THE
MAKER'S
DIET
REVOLUTION

THE
MAKER'S
DIET
REVOLUTION

THE *10 DAY* DIET
to Lose Weight and Detoxify Your Body, Mind, and Spirit

JORDAN RUBIN

Editorial assistance provided by Mike Yorkey (www.mikeyorkey.com)

DESTINY IMAGE® PUBLISHERS, INC.

P.O. Box 310, Shippensburg, PA 17257-0310

"Promoting Inspired Lives."

This book and all other Destiny Image, Revival Press, MercyPlace, Fresh Bread, Destiny Image Fiction, and Treasure House books are available at Christian bookstores and distributors worldwide.

For a U.S. bookstore nearest you, call 1-800-722-6774.

For more information on foreign distributors, call 717-532-3040.

Reach us on the Internet: www.destinyimage.com.

ISBN 13 HC: 978-0-7684-4228-1

ISBN 13 TP: 978-0-7684-0447-0

For Worldwide Distribution, Printed in the U.S.A.

1 2 3 4 5 6 7 8 / 17 16 15 14 13

IMPORTANT NOTICE FROM JORDAN RUBIN

This book is not intended to provide medical advice or to take the place of medical advice and treatment from your personal physician. Readers are advised to consult their own doctors or other qualified health professionals regarding treatment of their medical problems. Neither the publisher nor the author takes any responsibility for any possible consequences from any treatment, action, or application of medicine, supplement, herb, or preparation to any person reading or following the information in this book. If readers are taking prescription medications, they should consult with their physicians before beginning any nutrition or supplementation program.

In addition, below are governmental warnings regarding the consumption of raw eggs and raw juices:

- Consuming raw or undercooked eggs may increase your risk of food-borne illness.

- Juice that has not been pasteurized may contain bacteria that can increase the risk of food-borne illness. People most at risk are children, the elderly, and persons with a weakened immune system.

Related to the dietary supplements and foods discussed in this book: These statements have not been evaluated by the Foods and Drug Administration. This product is not intended to diagnose, treat, cure, or prevent any disease.

DISCLAIMERS REGARDING RAW DAIRY, RAW EGGS, RAW FISH, AND RAW JUICE

The following are government-issued warnings for the consumption of raw or undercooked foods and beverages.

- Raw milk products may contain disease-causing microorganisms. Persons at highest risk of disease from these organisms include newborns and infants, the elderly, pregnant women, those taking corticosteroids, antibiotics and antacids, and those having chronic illnesses and other conditions that weaken their immunity.

- Consuming raw or undercooked eggs may increase your risk of food-borne illness.

- Consuming raw or undercooked seafood may increase your risk of food-borne illness.

- Juice that has not been pasteurized may contain bacteria that can increase the risk of food-borne illness. People most at risk are children, the elderly, and persons with a weakened immune system.

Note: I am the founder of Beyond Organic and Garden of Life, and, where applicable, I am recommending these companies' products. Regarding other companies that I recommend, I do so because I consume their products and find them to be of good nutritional quality and taste. Beyond Organic and Garden of Life cannot be held responsible for the quality or claims of these products. Please do your research and consult with your healthcare practitioner prior to starting any new diet or supplement program.

CONTENTS

INTRODUCTION

If I mentioned the name Daniel in connection with the Bible, the first words most people would associate him with are "lion's den."

Sure, Daniel was thrown into a lair of hungry lions because he disobeyed a decree to bow and worship only King Darius when he was caught praying to the God of Abraham, Isaac, and Jacob. But it's what Daniel did long before he entered the lion's den that has always resonated with me.

When Daniel was in his teenage years, he was among the most handsome, physically fit, and intelligent young men in the royal line of Judah. Then disaster struck: King Nebuchadnezzar, the Babylonian ruler of the most powerful nation in the civilized world at the time, assembled a massive army to march into Jerusalem and to conquer the land in 605 B.C.

To demonstrate his dominance, King Nebuchadnezzar cherry-picked Jerusalem's best and brightest minds and most beautiful women as captives. Daniel, along with three young men his age—Hananiah, Misha-el, and Azariah—were carted off to Babylon, along with all of Judah's livestock and the Temple treasure.

There's every indication that this quartet was treated well because they were seen as assets by the King's court. They were the best of the best, the crème de la crème who would have gotten perfect 2400 scores on their SATs or aced their law school entrance exams today. Think National Merit Scholars.

Biblical academics believe this Fab Four was around fourteen years old when they were placed under the guidance of Ashpenaz, who was in charge of the palace personnel, to teach them the Chaldean language and literature.

Like hotshot recruits entering college, they were assigned the best foods from the King's own kitchen during their training period. Nothing would be spared for these elite scholars who looked—as well as acted—the part.

Daniel and his three friends may have grown up in spiritually depraved Judah, but somebody in their lives—a parent, an uncle, a rabbi, or a prophet—must have modeled how they should serve God. That's the best explanation I have for why they refused to eat the rich foods set before them at the King's table.

You see, these "foods" were considered detestable to the God of heaven whom they faithfully served. Perhaps they were presented with meats that had been sacrificed to idols, or meats that were unclean because the animals had been strangled or contaminated with blood or fat—or all of the above. More likely, though, they were offered meats that God forbade His people to eat in Leviticus 11 and Deuteronomy 14. I'm talking about pork, rabbits, camels, badgers, snakes, and flesh-eating birds such as vultures.

Shellfish was also unclean according to the ancient law, but it's doubtful that lobster or scampi were on King Nebuchadnezzar's menu because Babylon was too far away from a salt-water ocean. But they could have been served catfish, eel, or other smooth-skinned species that were also off limits according to God's commands.

Daniel also passed on the King's wine. While there was no scriptural injunction against drinking wine, perhaps Daniel knew the pitfalls that awaited those consuming excess alcohol and wanted to truly present his body to God as a living sacrifice. After all, the Babylonians were attempting to change his worldview by giving him a Chaldean education, to change his loyalty by giving him a new name (Daniel was called Belteschazzar, while Hananiah, Misha-el, and Azariah became the celebrated Shadrach, Meshach, and Abegnego who would later walk into the fiery furnace), and to change his lifestyle by giving him a new diet.

So, when presented with the King's banquet, Daniel politely inquired, *You got anything else to eat?*

When told no, he asked if he and his compatriots could consume a different diet that would be blessed by their God, which made Ashpenaz—in charge of their well-being—very nervous. He was afraid they would become pale and thin compared to the Babylonian youths in palace training. They wouldn't measure up. They'd fall behind.

"Give me and my buddies ten days," Daniel said. "That's all I ask. Let us eat only pulse and drink only water. If at the end of ten days we don't look better and look healthier than the young Babylonian men, then we'll eat the foods supplied by the King. Case closed."

I always marvel at the faith and courage it must have taken Daniel to risk his life for what he believed in. He simply was unwilling to dishonor God's commands, even in the area of diet.

Ashpenaz knew his head was on the chopping block if these four youths—the best of the best of Judah—became weaklings and lost their physical edge. When Daniel pressed his case, the steward reluctantly agreed to their experiment. The four could eat their pulse—the ripe, edible seeds and produce of a wide range of plants—and drink only water for ten days.

In a sense, Daniel was placing his life on the line as well, but he was willing to put God's principles for healthy eating to the test. The story goes that for ten days they ate only pulse and drank only water. At the end of their experiment, they were found to be greater in health and excelled in wisdom and mental acuity and clarity when compared to their Babylonian counterparts. No one was smarter, better looking, or healthier than Daniel, Hananiah, Misha-el, and Azariah.

Based on the objective results of following their "Maker's Diet," the four young Hebrews were allowed to continue consuming a diet approved by God for the balance of the three-year training program. Scripture tells us that when they were examined by King Nebuchadnezzar himself, they were found to be "ten times better" in health, wisdom, and understanding than the leading young men of Babylon who had received the same education.

Ten times better? When you stop and think about it, that was quite a feat back then and would be a massive advantage today. One-hundredth of a second—comparable to the length of a fingernail in this case—was the difference between Michael Phelps coming home from the 2008 Beijing Olympic Games with a record eight gold medals versus seven golds and one silver around his neck. Likewise, the blink of an eye is often the difference between winning a sprint to the finish line in a bike race, on the 400-meter running track, at a speed-skating rink, or in the swimming pool. Victory in sport is always a tiny differential of far less than 1 percent.

Yet Daniel and his three friends were "ten times better," which is almost like lapping the field in a middle-distance running race. Imagine if you were found to be ten times the student, ten times the teacher, ten times more effective as an attorney, ten times more proficient in sales, ten times more precise as a surgeon, or ten times stronger and faster than the competition. Think of the advantage you would have over everyone.

In other words, imagine that you were LeBron James for a moment. Okay, I'm exaggerating, but sometimes when I see LeBron take over an NBA basketball game in the waning moments, I can imagine what it's like for someone to be clearly head and shoulders above the competition. That's what Daniel must have been like against his competition in the palace court. He was ten times better, which is why the King gave him more and more responsibilities.

The author of the Book of Daniel was Daniel himself. This was his story, and the Spirit of God inspired his words. Compared to some of the other miraculous events described in the book—interpreting King Nebuchadnezzar's dreams; Shadrach, Meshach, and Abednego walking in and out of the roaring flames inside the furnace; Daniel surviving without a scratch in a den of hungry lions; and seeing astounding visions from God Himself—I still believe that Daniel's steadfast faith and the fact that he and his friends excelled to the point of being "ten times better" than other young men in the palace court is the greatest miracle recounted in the Book of Daniel.

WHY DANIEL RESONATES TODAY

Another reason why I identify with Daniel's amazing journey of faith is because I wasn't much older than he was when I faced a similar life-changing choice:

At the age of nineteen, do I follow the conventional wisdom on how to treat several incurable diseases that jeopardized my life? Or do I follow God's plan for good health set forth in the Bible?

I had just finished my freshman year at Florida State University when I took a counselor position at a summer church camp. Out of nowhere, I was hit with nausea, stomach cramps, high fever, and horrible digestive problems. That was the first wave; the follow-up was a tsunami of violent diarrhea that knocked me for a loop and sapped any remaining energy I had. I would drop twenty pounds from my already lean frame in just six days at camp.

My health deteriorated over the next few months, and I was forced to withdraw from college at the start of my sophomore year. I went back home to Palm Beach Gardens, Florida, where my parents knew something was seriously wrong. When my fever spiked to 105 degrees, they immediately stepped into action, filling our bathtub with ice and cold water. My father gently eased my fever-ridden body into the chilly bathwater, but I was close to incoherent.

My parents rushed me to the local hospital, where specialists and medical technicians conducted various tests, including a sigmoidoscopy and an upper GI series that allowed them to examine the condition in my intestinal tract and look for any irregularities.

I was examined by a gastroenterologist, who recognized the symptoms of high fever, night sweats, loss of appetite, general feeling of weakness, severe abdominal cramps, and diarrhea—often bloody—as symptoms of inflammatory bowel disease. After running a battery of diagnostic tests, the doctor delivered a stunning verdict: I was stricken with a digestive ailment known as Crohn's disease.

"How do we treat it?" I asked.

"There's no known cure," replied the gastroenterologist. "You'll probably be on powerful anti-inflammatory and immunosuppressives for the rest of your life. You could be facing surgery to remove parts of your small intestine and potentially your colon."

My doctor then rattled off words such as "resection" and "colectomy" and "ostomy." None of those terms were familiar to me, and later I would learn what they really meant: I would have to live with the surgical removal of my colon and wear bags to collect fecal waste from my body. To a nineteen-year-old preparing to find his way in the world, that sounded like a fate worse than death.

Neither my parents nor I liked that scenario, so we set out on a path that would take me to sixty-nine doctors, medical practitioners, and health experts and attempt treatments ranging from conventional medicine to "natural cures." We tapped every medical and nutritional mind we could, and I personally read more than three hundred books on health and nutrition. I tried every possible diet out there in my attempt to leave no stone unturned.

Nothing stopped the death spiral that my health was in. I lost nearly half of my body weight and was reduced to 104 pounds, a frightfully thin figure who resembled a concentration camp survivor. The medical team treating me prepared my parents for the news that I might not make it.

I'll never forget the night in my hospital room when nurses, phlebotomists, and doctors desperately tried to get an IV in me to rehydrate my shriveled body. After one failed attempt, a nurse ran out of my hospital room. I overheard her say, "This young man isn't going to make it until the next morning."

I truly believed this was it for me. I was ready to die and go home to be with the Lord. After four hours of agony, they successfully inserted a needle into my vein.

I woke up the next morning alive, but I was far from healed. When my condition stabilized, I was sent home with a half-dozen medications to deal with the stabbing pains in my gut, and I made dozens of trips to the bathroom each day.

It was about that time when I made a commitment to God. "Lord, if you heal me and I come out of this alive," I prayed, "and if I can help just one person overcome a horrific disease like mine, this living hell will have all been worth it."

I also took a major step of faith in asking my mother to take my picture. She was reluctant to do so and even asked me if she could wait to take the photo when I looked better. I demanded she take the picture now, as I wanted the world to see what God was about to do in my life.

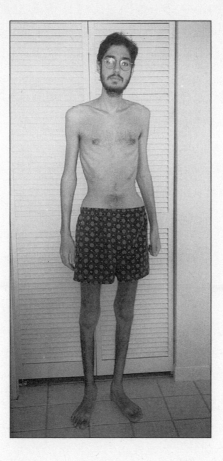

Despite my step of faith, my health continued to deteriorate. The medical doctors counseled my parents that it was time for me to go under the knife. Feeling like I was out of options, I consented to life-altering ostomy surgery.

Just before the surgical plan was enacted, my father was introduced by phone to a San Diego nutritionist who offered to show me God's health plan in the Bible. He believed I could be healed if I followed a diet based on the Bible, proven through history and confirmed by science.

I had nothing to lose, and better yet, I believed that this may be God's plan to heal me. I boarded a plane to travel across the country in my wheelchair. Upon my arrival in San Diego, I feasted on the Word of God and followed an eating plan that I would later call the "Maker's Diet."

After forty days, I added twenty-nine much-needed pounds and soon topped 150 pounds for the first time in nearly two years. Six weeks later, I was back to my old weight and ready to begin my life again.

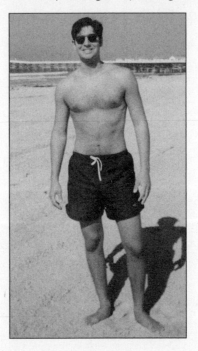

Not only did I get well without medication or surgery, but I was inspired to transform the health of this nation and world one life at a time. Upon returning home to South Florida, I worked at a health food store where I shared my story and encouraged many customers to change their diet. A few short months later, I started a health and nutrition company, Garden of Life, that in the following decade would become the most popular nutritional supplement company in American health food stores.

During this time, I've been able to share my life-changing experiences and what I learned about healthy living in seminars spanning the globe as well as in major media—television, radio, magazine, and newspapers. I hosted an international television program and would go on to write more than twenty books on nutrition, health, and wellness, including *The Maker's Diet*, which released in 2004 and today has over 2 million copies in print.

In 2009, I was led to purchase thousands of acres of farmland, sources of pure spring water, heirloom seeds, and livestock with genetics resembling those found in biblical times. Taking nutrition a step "beyond" organic is a recently realized but longtime passion of mine that has resulted in a focused mission to provide people with the world's healthiest foods, beverages, skin and body care, and living nutritional supplements. My ultimate goal is see one million people living beyond organic by the year 2020.

During the last decade and a half, I have studied with and learned from some of the greatest minds in medicine, nutrition, and sustainable agriculture. Additionally, I have successfully coached thousands of people to transform their health as I had.

But perhaps my greatest nutritional revelation occurred at the end of 2012 while on a mission trip to India. On a long drive back from a remote city in the state of Andra Pradesh, the Lord spoke to me and laid out the diet plan that you'll read about in this book, *The Maker's Diet Revolution*.

I believe this new plan, which expands upon the principles found in the original *Maker's Diet*, will create a health and wellness revolution in the lives of millions of people.

NEXT GENERATION

In the following pages of *The Maker's Diet Revolution*, I'll expand on three principles, or pillars, of biblical health. They are:

1. Eat what God created for food.

2. Don't alter God's design.

3. Don't let any food or drink become your idol.

The inspiration for these three principles comes from Rex Russell, M.D., author of *What the Bible Says About Healthy Living*. Dr. Russell was a mentor and a good friend of mine right up until his death in 2009.

The truth is that the Bible has a definition of food and a definition of filth. This is clearly laid out in Leviticus 11 and Deuteronomy 14 as it pertains to animal foods. In addition, there are many items in our modern diet that are made exclusively of laboratory-created chemicals. These are clearly *not* part of the Creator's eating plan. God did, however, create—for us to enjoy—wonderful foods that are teeming with nutrients, beneficial compounds, and best of all, great taste.

Not altering God's design has to do with how food is grown, raised, processed, and prepared. For plant foods, I'm referring to what we do before seeds are planted in the ground, while the food is growing, and after the food is harvested.

Let's talk about how food starts in the fields. The rise of Big Agriculture in the last century means that fewer and fewer farmers are growing more and more food on larger and larger plots of land. To increase crop yields and to get the most of their acreage, large-scale farming operations plant seeds containing genetically modified organisms (GMOs) that are resistant to insect infestation.

If you've heard of genetically modified foods but are not sure what they are, you should know that these crops have been genetically engineered using the latest molecular biological techniques. In other words, these seeds were modified in the laboratory by taking genes from one organism and inserting them into another to make them grow higher, larger, denser, and more resistant to pests.

The problem is that we're using molecular engineering to force genetic information across the protective species barrier in an unnatural way. While the idea of creating pest-resistant plant species is laudable, the problem is that scientists have successfully added genes to foods that weren't originally part of that food's creation, which changes the DNA of the crop.

As of this date, these laboratory-created mutations have not been subjected to any sort of rigorous testing on humans, but genetically modified foods have been linked to toxic and allergic reactions causing sickness and sterility in livestock, which is why they are banned as food ingredients in Europe and other nations. Even though we don't have scientific studies outlining just how detrimental the short-term or long-term effects will be, we do know that GMO crops demand higher levels of toxic herbicides and pesticides, which go straight into the food you eat—and straight into your stomach and ultimately your bloodstream.

Bottom line: GMO foods offer no benefits, only health risks. But if you're like most people, you're probably unknowingly exposing yourself to these excessive toxins sneaked into your food. Stop being a victim today.

Another form of altering God's design is hybridization, which is taking two species from the same plant family and grafting them together. In the animal world, we would call this selective breeding, but in the plant world, you're basically creating a new species.

A prime example of hybridization would be seedless watermelons, which were created in the laboratory by a Japanese scientist who figured out that pollinating plants with a normal complement of chromosomes with a plant genetically modified with *double* the number of chromosomes would produce a fruit that lacked seeds.

What's more is that watermelon patches and every other conventional crop are subjected to pesticides and herbicides to battle insects and pests that damage the crops. Crop-duster planes routinely douse crops with chemicals that are toxic, resulting in a less healthy food supply. In addition, synthetic fertilizers used to replenish soil fertility may stimulate rapid plant growth, but they bring along unintended consequences. These fertilizers are made up of nitrogen salts, which return little, if any, vital minerals to the soil and actually cause micronutrient imbalances. Thus, the nutritive value of foods grown in our soils has declined significantly in the last hundred years.

The use of pesticides and herbicides extends to the meat and dairy we eat as well. These days, cattle, chickens, and "farm-raised" fish are fattened on feed containing unhealthy chemicals as well as antibiotics that are added to compensate for the unsanitary and deplorable living conditions on factory farms. To add insult to injury, the majority of U.S. livestock are loaded with hormones and growth promotants that contaminate meat and dairy—a practice that can lead to serious health challenges in humans, especially children and teenagers.

Another example of how we alter God's design for food is the way the "genius of man" has figured how to prepare, manufacture, cook, microwave, and market mass-produced foods in ways that are terribly unhealthy for us. Too many of the so-called foods sold in our nation's supermarkets are not really food because they are made from synthetic and processed ingredients to produce a more competitively priced product with a longer shelf life. These ingredients have been stripped clean of nutrients and pumped up with additives and preservatives. I'm talking about vegetable oils, frozen pizza, ice cream, processed cheese, potato chips, cookie dough, white bread, dinner rolls, snack foods, doughnuts, candy, salad dressing, margarine, and much more. The list is endless.

The final principle—to not let any food or drink become your idol—refers to how we are addicted to foods and beverages in the American culture. It doesn't matter if you're a churchgoer or not, but we're a people who eat early and eat often. We wake up and march like zombies, either to the kitchen to make coffee or driving to a local coffee shop. We sit down to big breakfasts with eggs, pancakes, sausage, and hash browns; enjoy bacon deluxe burgers and fries at lunch; and dine on hubcap-sized platters of food in the evening. And then there's snacking on chips and cookies before and after meals.

Sugar or salt, we love them both, and caffeine—well, it can be considered the most widely abused drug in the world. Coffee is the most popular beverage in the United States—even above bottled water. On average, Americans drink 400 cups of coffee annually. As overwhelming as that number is, it's nothing compared to our need for a salty snack or a sugar fix.

For many, life is justifying the next ice cream.

Got a promotion? Go get an ice cream to celebrate.

Got laid off? Get an ice cream to make you feel better.

Our addiction to food means we are consuming too many calories and chemicals that our bodies can't handle. Something has to give, and, unfortunately, it's our health.

I believe it's critical to return to our Maker's plan for eating healthy. We are God's temple, and He cares about us and what we eat and what we do. He wants us to live long, healthy lives so that we can be beacons of light to a lost generation for as long as we can.

That can happen if you follow the Maker's Diet Revolution eating plan.

FORGOTTEN SECRETS

The Maker's Diet Revolution eating plan embraces the body's natural cycles by employing the ancient strategy of regular cleansing and building.

When it comes to health, there are only two governing principles, which are agreed upon by virtually every health expert:

1. *Get the good in*, meaning we must get nutrients into the appropriate cells of the body's organs and tissues.

2. *Get the bad out*, meaning we need to stimulate the excretion of toxins out of the body.

These twin goals can be accomplished by *cleansing*, which is the body's way to rid itself of toxins, and *building*, which is the body's way to create and effectively restore healthy organs, tissues, bloodstream, lymphatic system, and digestive tract, building strength within the body and fortifying a defense system against invaders such as toxins.

I will devote the first part of *The Maker's Diet Revolution* to *cleansing the body*.

The cleansing process is the key to a healthy body, and we were created to undergo a specific cycle of cleansing and building to break down waste and to build up strength. If you look back into history at the natural health experts of the past—even to the father of Western medicine, Hippocrates—they all said that removing waste from the body is the starting point for good health.

Cleansing is not something you do every once in a while. Cleansing is something the body does every day, whether you like it or not or whether you cooperate or not. That said, cleansing comes in many forms. You may not realize this, but what we call the common cold—congestion and mucus expulsion—is the body's proactive reaction, ridding itself of germs and invaders and a form of cleansing.

The Maker's Diet Revolution will put you on the fast track to experiencing the many benefits of cleansing, which will be accomplished quarterly, monthly, weekly, and even daily following the ancient traditions of the world's healthiest people.

Building up the body is the second pillar of The Maker's Diet Revolution as well as the second part of this program. You build your body by fortifying the body's "terrain" or transforming the internal environment.

Toxins can't live in a healthy body with a healthy terrain. This explains why five people can go to a restaurant, order a large fish entrée to be served family style at the table, and three get sick from ingesting an overabundance of bacteria while two were okay.

Since they ate the same fish, why were some doubling over in pain two hours later and some were sleeping just fine?

The difference was their terrain.

RAISING YOUR LEVEL OF HEALTH

Activating and optimizing the cleansing-and-building cycle within your body is the reason I'm confident that your journey on *The Maker's Diet Revolution* will create a transformation in your health and in the health of your family. In fact, I wouldn't be surprised if after following the Maker's Diet Revolution nutrition program your body is flooded with a level of health that is "ten times better" than others your age—similar to what Daniel experienced over 2,600 years ago.

After Daniel and his buddies passed their ten-day test, God gave Daniel, Hananiah, Misha-el, and Azariah great ability to learn over the next three years, which allowed them to master all the science and literature at the time. God also gave Daniel the special ability to understand the meanings of dreams and visions.

We're told in Scripture that Daniel and all the young men had to pass their oral exams before they could become part of the king's palace court. King Nebuchadnezzar conducted their final exams in long conversations with the young men, and none of them impressed him as much as Daniel, Hananiah, Misha-el, and Azariah, who were immediately placed on his regular staff of advisors.

> *Whenever the king consulted them in any matter requiring wisdom*
> *and balanced judgment, he found them ten times more capable than*

any of the magicians and enchanters in his entire kingdom (Daniel 1:20 NLT).

How would you like to be ten times greater in health and wisdom than any and all of your contemporaries and to take every area of your life to the next level?

If you carefully follow the instructions detailed in the pages to come, I believe you can and you will. Best of all, your journey can begin today.

Welcome to the Revolution!

Part I

CLEANSING YOUR BODY

1

YOUR REVOLUTION STARTS
WITH A 10-DAY CLEANSE

Talk about sensory overload.

Sari-clad women rode sidesaddle on dusty scooters as their husbands took daring risks through chaotic intersections, turbaned men propelled bicycle-powered rickshaws with entire families in tow, and dark smoke from exhaust-spewing three-wheeled taxis blackened the sky as our transport vehicle weaved its way past roadside markets and tin-roofed lean-tos.

Welcome to the colorful sights and pungent smells of southeastern India. It was early December 2012, and our group was traveling from Srikakulam, a crowded, extremely depressed city of 2.7 million, back to our hotel in Visakhapatnam—called Vizag for short—following an evangelistic crusade presented by my good friend, Dr. Pete Sulack, a chiropractor from Knoxville, Tennessee, and an international evangelist and president of Matthew 10 International Ministries.

I don't care much for international travel. That's actually putting it mildly. As someone who's dealt with huge digestive issues in the past, traveling halfway around the world to a place where people strongly encourage you not to drink the water, eat the food, or open your mouth when taking a shower makes traveling to Third World countries problematic for me.

I did my due diligence on the region I was heading to, although I wish someone had told me that bathrooms typically don't come equipped with toilet paper and many homes lacked toilets period. At any rate, I packed an arsenal of nutritional supplements that included probiotics and digestive enzymes. I brought along several homeopathic remedies to battle everything from dysentery to puncture wounds to even malaria. I also stowed away a ten-day supply of superfood snacks that we had recently developed at Beyond Organic called EA Live Foods.

EA stands for "enzyme-activated," a process that renders foods highly digestible and packed with nutrients. My favorite staples were EA Live Granola and EA Live Seven Seed Crackers as well as sprouted almonds, pumpkin seeds, pecans, cashews, cinnamon pecans, and chocolate walnuts.

Fortunately on most days, I was able to consume one good healthy meal at a nice hotel or restaurant in Vizag, but when our evangelistic team went on the road, I relied on my stash of EA Live foods and healthy snacks to get me through the day.

I traveled to India as part of the Matthew 10 ministry team spearheaded by Dr. Pete Sulack, whose great-grandparents risked their lives nearly a century ago to take the Gospel to the headhunters of Nagaland, a state in the far northeastern part of India. Christianity spread like wildfire among the Naga tribes, who left the old tribal customs and brutal traditions—such as preserving the heads of their enemies as trophies—for new cultural and spiritual practices. Today, more than 95 percent of the Naga people claim to be Christians.

Here is the fascinating twist to this story: churches in Nagaland were praying that a descendent of Dr. Sulack's great-grandparents would return to India to evangelize souls. When Dr. Pete heard about this, it confirmed in his heart that the Lord was calling him to India to win a billion souls for the Gospel.

Dr. Pete has been making annual crusades to India since 2005. When he visited our home to describe his exciting work, he looked at me and my wife, Nicki, and said, "You're welcome to join us on our next trip."

I could tell Nicki was extremely interested in taking Dr. Pete up on his offer. After he left for the evening, Nicki said to me, "We're going!"

There was no way I could deny her or the way God was leading us to India, so I signed on as well. As for my concern about the food and cleanliness of India, I knew the trip wouldn't be easy, but I also knew God had a plan for that, too.

Meanwhile, my eight-year-old son Joshua was in the midst of a spiritual awakening at that time. He had eight dreams over an eleven-day period and described one of them to Nicki as she was driving him home from school.

"Mom, I had a dream last night, and God told me that we're going to India."

Nicki nearly drove out of her lane, then caught herself. Neither of us had mentioned to Joshua or his two younger siblings that we were going to India. The trip was still eight months away, and India wasn't a normal dinner table conversation in our household.

"Who's we?" she asked.

"Me, you, and Dad."

"Well, Joshua, your father and I *are* going to India. We're planning to go on a gospel crusade with an evangelistic team just after Thanksgiving."

"Who are you going with?"

"Dr. Pete Sulack."

Joshua nodded. He'd met Dr. Pete before as well as his four sons—two of whom were close to Joshua's age. They had spent some time together a few months earlier.

"Well, I'm going, too."

"But you don't have a passport," Nicki said.

"Then let's get me one."

Nicki and I had never planned on bringing our eight-year-old to a Third World country, where we would be concerned not only for his health, but also for his safety. When you bring together large crowds and preach the Gospel in a land dominated by Hinduism (80 percent of the country)—with Islam making inroads (12 percent of the populace)—things could get dicey.

After Nicki told me about their conversation, we discussed what we should do. We then prayed about the decision. When we felt the leading of the Lord to have Joshua join us, I knew we had to ask Dr. Pete if that would be okay. No young child had ever been part of his international crusades, so Joshua would be the first.

When we made the request to bring Joshua, Dr. Pete smiled. "We'd be honored to have him," he said.

The long journey from South Florida to southeastern India was grueling—more than twenty-seven hours en route—but what a rich and rewarding experience for the three of us. Joshua was a welcome addition to our twelve-person group during our prayer and worship meetings. He witnessed four evangelistic rallies before audiences that numbered 20,000 people on the first night and more than 80,000 the last night. He saw thousands saved and healed, and he heard me testify to God's healing power to 80,000 Srikakulamians at an outdoor field teeming with people as far as the eye could see.

While returning from the awe-inspiring evangelistic event in Srikakulam, I was lost in my thoughts as our car motored along. I glanced outside at the dark Indian countryside and felt I heard the Lord's voice. He said, *Jordan, I know this was a big sacrifice for you to come to India.*

Yes, there was the commitment of time and money, and the Lord knew I had grave concerns about traveling so far and my difficulties adjusting to foreign lands. I had some rough experiences while in Indonesia and South Africa—even in a Western country such as Australia.

But Nicki felt called to go. Joshua really wanted to join us in India as well. Even though I had a lot of personal trepidation, I knew we were supposed to be part of Dr. Pete's Matthew 10 team.

AN OUTLINE FOR THE DANIEL DIET

It was rewarding to watch how the Lord was moving in the subcontinent of India. We witnessed thousands receive Christ as their Savior, and I saw people run to the altar when Dr. Pete invited them to follow Jesus and receive all that He had waiting for them. I saw Indian people healed of diseases, released from addictions, and set free from demons tormenting their souls. Quite frankly, I had never witnessed anything like it, and I was humbled by the transforming power of God.

And then I heard His voice again while in the car driving back to our hotel:

Because you have honored Me by coming all the way to India, I am going to honor you by giving you an innovative idea and strategy to transform the health of My people each and every night of the crusade.

"Really, Lord?" I whispered.

Really.

I received the idea for the Daniel Diet on the night of the first crusade, as well as several other unique nutritional concepts during my trip. The Lord gave me the outline for an authentic, ten-day partial fasting program consisting of the foods and beverage similar to what Daniel and his three friends consumed some 2,600 years ago:

> *Prove thy servants, I beseech thee, ten days; and let them give us pulse to eat, and water to drink* (Daniel 1:12 ASV).

Upon my return to Florida, I couldn't wait to start formulating what I would call the Daniel Diet. I researched the definition of "pulse" and discovered that pulse consists of all leguminous plants. Pulse is nutrient-dense and high in fiber; contains beneficial fatty acids, vitamins, and minerals; contains no cholesterol; has a low glycemic index; and is high in protein. Examples of pulse would be fruits, vegetables, nuts, seeds, beans, and grains.

I enlisted my team at Beyond Organic to help me create three blends of nutrient-dense pulse that people could consume exclusively during a ten-day period. Next, I decided to test the idea. It just so happened that each year in January, the congregation my family has attended for the last four years, Generation Church in nearby Jupiter, invited me to speak on the topic of fasting. Six weeks after getting back from India, I preached on the benefits of fasting and laid out the foundation for the Daniel Diet.

I shared the story of Daniel and invited the church members to join me on a Daniel Diet where we would eat only pulse and drink only water for ten days, commit to pray corporately three times per day on conference calls, and meet each evening for a time of worship, teaching, and prayer. I made a similar offer to a select group of leaders at Beyond Organic, the vertically integrated farm-to-family nutrition company I founded in 2009.

As I write these words, there have been over four hundred people who have championed the Daniel Diet. Together, we consumed only EA Pulse—a nutrient-dense blend of raw and/or sprouted organic fruits, veggies, nuts, seeds, legumes, and herbs—and drank only structured water.

The results of the Daniel Diet were unexpected and unbelievable.

We had one individual lose 24 pounds in just ten days. I lost 19 pounds, which was shocking since I'm not overweight and carry only a small amount of body fat. I went from 193 pounds to 174 lean and mean pounds.

We saw dozens of men lose 15, 13, and 11 pounds. We had women lose 11 or 10 pounds in ten days. Nicki, who's thin to begin with, lost eight pounds. My children even went on the Daniel Diet, and even though they did not lose weight or even need to lose weight, they were more energetic, had clearer skin, zero nasal congestion, improvements in behavior, and slept great.

While these results were extraordinary, the average reported weight loss for male participants in the ten-day Daniel Diet was 14.5 pounds, and the average weight loss for female participants was 8.3 pounds. This is truly remarkable considering that each participant consumed between 1,200 and 1,500 nutrient-dense calories daily.

These results defy the common understanding that in order to lose weight you must greatly reduce calories. As I mentioned, a diet of EA Pulse is close to 1,500 calories a day, a number that has historically been shown to result in weight loss averaging 1 pound a week. Yet we had plenty of folks losing weight at a rate nearly ten times faster!

That's why I've decided to make the 10-Day Daniel Diet the centerpiece of the Maker's Diet Revolution program. I believe when you experience these incredible results for yourself, you'll be compelled to share your experience with others who will do the same.

This will be the start of a health revolution in your life, your family, your church, your city, your state, and our nation.

TEN DAYS TO TRANSFORM YOUR LIFE

I know a lot of people talk about fasting and cleansing and there are stacks of books out there on these topics, but I believe there is something supernatural about committing ten days of your life to eating the best of God's creation, drinking the water provided from heaven, and spending time in prayer and meditation on the Word of God.

For the first time in more than 2,600 years, you are going to unlock the cleansing secret from the Bible and experience a radical transformation in body, mind, and spirit. Ever since the Lord gave me the outline for this ten-day program, I've been recommending the Daniel Diet to people all over the world who are desperately in need of a health transformation, and their testimonies are compelling to say the least.

If you have ten days to devote to your health and want to treat your body to the ultimate cleanse and detoxification program, this would be it. The Daniel Diet is a way to cleanse your body while experiencing the miracle of fasting, so don't delay. Make tomorrow the first day of your own health revolution!

THE DANIEL DIET

The Daniel Diet is a partial fast involving the consumption of *only* water and pulse for ten days, the seeking of God's face in daily prayer three set times per day, and daily Bible study and learning.

The Daniel Diet is based on the first chapter of the Book of Daniel, which describes how Daniel and three young compatriots from Judah were taken into captivity. Instead of consuming the king's delicacies, they asked to consume only foods that the God of Abraham, Isaac, and Jacob had blessed. Paraphrasing from the New King James version, we learn this:

> Please test your servants for ten days, and let them give us pulse to eat and water to drink. Then let our appearance be examined before you.... Then at the end of the ten days, their features appeared better and healthier than all the young men who ate a portion of the king's delicacies.... As for these four youths, God gave them learning and skill in all literature and wisdom.

According to my understanding of the Hebrew definition of pulse, I have created what I believe to be an authentic Daniel Diet.

WHY FAST?

The Daniel Diet gives you many of the benefits of fasting but is much easier and simpler to follow and doesn't come with the potential dangers of going without food.

Now you may be asking *why* it's important to fast.

The answers are numerous, but the main reason to fast, in my opinion, is to receive breakthrough in areas of your life that nothing else can bring and to open doors that cannot be opened by anything else. God reveals this in Isaiah:

> Is this not the fast that I have chosen: to loose the bonds of wickedness, to undo the heavy burdens, to let the oppressed go free, and that you break every yoke?...Then your light shall break forth like the morning, your healing shall spring forth speedily, and your righteousness shall go before you.... (Isaiah 58:6,8).

Look at these incredible spiritual benefits of fasting:

1. Fasting can bring you closer to God.

2. Fasting can make you more sensitive to God's voice.

3. Fasting helps break addictions.

4. Fasting shows us our weakness and allows us to rely on God's strength.

Paracelsus, the famed 15th-century physician and alchemist who believed in the body's ability to heal itself, said fasting activates "the Healer within." Here are some of the incredible emotional benefits of fasting:

1. Fasting helps support healthy emotions.

2. Fasting clears your mind of negative thoughts.

3. Fasting can bring peace.

"There is not a habit or weakness that can survive a siege of prayer and fasting," Edward Earle Purinton wrote in his book, *The Philosophy of Fasting*.

And finally, here are twelve physical benefits of fasting:

1. Fasting helps break addictions to junk food, drinking, and smoking.

2. Fasting supports the body's detoxification systems.

3. Fasting promotes healthy weight loss.

4. Fasting promotes healthy energy levels.

5. Fasting supports healthy aging, healthy skin, and a glowing complexion.

6. Fasting promotes healthy memory, focus, and concentration.

7. Fasting reduces stress and promotes sound sleep.

8. Fasting supports cardiovascular health.

9. Fasting promotes healthy digestion and elimination.

10. Fasting supports healthy inflammation response and promotes joint comfort.

11. Fasting supports healthy immune system function.

12. Fasting promotes healthy hormonal balance.

Dr. Otto H.F. Buchinger, who supervised more than 70,000 fasts, once said, "Fasting is…a royal road to healing for anyone who agrees to take it for the transformation of body, mind, and spirit."

WHAT IS DANIEL'S CHALLENGE?

In Babylon, Daniel and his friends requested a diet of pulse and water rather than the king's "delicacies." After ten days, the king found them healthier and stronger. After three years, he found them ten times better in countenance (health) and wisdom than the most learned in the kingdom, as we read in Daniel 1:

The Battle of Fasting

Whenever you start a fast, keep this admonition found in Ephesians 6:12 (NIV) in mind: "For our struggle is not against flesh and blood, but against the rulers, against the authorities, against the powers of this dark world and against the spiritual forces of evil in the heavenly realms."

You need to be aware that the enemy knows that if you undertake a fast, then you are about to see an incredible break-through in your life, and he wants to stop it. Here are some of the challenges that you may face during your ten-day Daniel Diet:

On the spiritual side:

- Circumstances in your life may seem to be impossible to overcome; this means the fast is working.

- Temptation to break the fast may seem to increase, and you may come up with several "good" reasons to stop it. This means the fast is working.

On the emotional side:

- Because your body will begin throwing off deadly emotions, an initial increase in nervousness, anxiety, and worry may result. This means the fast is working.

On the physical side:

- Since your body will begin to detoxify, you may experience a coated tongue, headaches, bad breath, body odor, digestion and elimination changes, fatigue, and even the sniffles. This means the fast is working.

The king assigned them a daily amount of food and wine from the king's table. They were to be trained for three years, and after that they were to enter the king's service.

Among those who were chosen were some from Judah: Daniel, Hananiah, Mishael and Azariah. ...But Daniel resolved not to defile himself with the royal food and wine, and he asked the chief official for permission not to defile himself this way.

Now God had caused the official to show favor and compassion to Daniel, but the official told Daniel, "I am afraid of my lord the king, who has assigned your food and drink. Why should he see you looking worse than the other young men your age? The king would then have my head because of you."

Daniel then said to the guard whom the chief official had appointed over Daniel, Hananiah, Mishael and Azariah, "Please test your servants for ten days: Give us nothing but vegetables [pulse] to eat and water to drink. Then compare our appearance with that of the young men who eat the royal food, and treat your servants in accordance with what you see." So he agreed to this and tested them for ten days (Daniel 1:5-6, 8-13 NIV).

Ten days later:

At the end of the ten days they looked healthier and better nourished than any of the young men who ate the royal food (Daniel 1:15 NIV).

Three years later:

So the guard took away their choice food and the wine they were to drink and gave them vegetables instead. To these four young men God gave knowledge and understanding of all kinds of literature and learning. And Daniel could understand visions and dreams of all kinds.

At the end of the time set by the king to bring them into his service, the chief official presented them to Nebuchadnezzar. The king talked with them, and he found none equal to Daniel, Hananiah, Mishael and Azariah; so they entered the king's service. In every matter of wisdom and understanding about which the king questioned them, he found them ten times better than all the magicians and enchanters in his whole kingdom (Daniel 1:16-20 NIV).

Daniel experienced great short-term health results by following the diet that now bears his name, but his long-term health was evidenced by the fact that he outlived King Nebuchadnezzar and was alert and coherent enough to advise the King's grandson, Belshazzar, roughly seventy years after the reign of Nebuchadnezzar began. Now *that's* a telling piece of information! (See Daniel Chapter 5.)

It seems like such a silly thing for Daniel to have requested a different diet, especially considering his circumstances. How many of us would have happily preferred the delicacies of the king? We see, however, that the four young men who ate the diet of pulse and water were given abundant health, great knowledge, and skill in all learning and wisdom by God.

Daniel risked his life for a diet that later provided him a cutting edge above all of the wise men and counselors in the kingdom. Daniel provides us a valuable lesson about how our health and even our intellectual ability—throughout our lives—are dependent on our choice of diet.

Why not give Daniel's diet a chance to help you?

THE 10-DAY DANIEL DIET

You can follow the Daniel Diet in one of two recommended ways.

Option Number 1

Purchase fresh raw fruits, vegetables, nuts, and seeds (organic is preferable) from your local health food or grocery store and consume as outlined below.

You begin by drinking a half-liter of water not long after you wake up. Then be sure to pray at 9 A.M. or at a morning time that's suitable for you.

Your first of three meals is at 12:30 P.M., which consists of one kind of fruit along with healthy fats from avocado, nuts, and seeds and/or coconut. Try to consume only one fruit (two pieces if allowed) and if possible, alternate different fruits each day.

Then some time in the afternoon, approximately 3 P.M., take time to pray, if possible.

At 3:30 P.M., you're going to consume a veggie meal combined with a good source of healthy fats. You can choose any combination of raw veggies. For example, multiple veggies are allowed and should be combined with healthy, high-fat foods such as avocado, coconut (mature, young, or Thai), or raw soaked and sprouted nuts and seeds such as almonds. Fibrous veggies, such as broccoli or cauliflower, can be lightly cooked, although I prefer that you eat your veggies raw if possible.

Can you make a salad? Sure, but since the Daniel Diet nixes the consumption of salt, oils, and sweeteners, this eliminates salad dressings. If you want to make a salad, the way to do it is to toss together greens and add cucumbers, peppers, celery and onions. Then in a blender, throw in avocado, add some chopped onions, raw lemon juice, sliced tomatoes, and hit the power button. What you'll produce is a cross between a dressing, a salad, and a soup. Kind of like a super guacamole, which is delicious on top of your veggies.

At 6:30 P.M., repeat a raw fruit and healthy fat meal with one type of fruit and healthy fats from avocado, coconut, and raw soaked and sprouted nuts and seeds. Throughout the day, make sure to consume between 100 to 128 ounces of pure water per day. This will help facilitate the body's cleansing process.

Please note that I recommend you skip the traditional breakfast meal and start eating at what would be considered after lunch time each day while following the Daniel Diet. The reasoning for this will be explained in greater detail in Chapter 2 in the section entitled "Daily Cleansing."

While you may be used to consuming a large meal shortly upon waking, I believe by narrowing your daily eating time window and thus lengthening your fasting and cleansing time, your health will greatly improve in many ways.

What Others Are Saying About the Daniel Diet

We asked those who participated in the Daniel Diet program to document what they did and share their results with us. Here are a few testimonials:

During the Daniel Diet, I prayed a lot and I think that helped me to stay focused. I believe the Daniel Diet was very helpful and caused me to be disciplined both spiritually and physically. I lost a total of 24 pounds and three inches from my waist.

—FRANK M.

I was stunned and amazed at how God worked through the Daniel Diet. I have fasted before, but never have I had such clarity of mind. I felt great and got many, many compliments on my skin while losing a total of 10 pounds.

God proved His faithfulness during the Daniel Diet and showed me once again His complete love for me and that He will *never* leave me nor forsake me!

—CECILIA B.

I have lost a total 15 pounds and have had no lightheadedness, no dizziness, no headaches, no aches of any kind, and no problems with vision or cognitive function. In fact, I've experienced increased mental clarity, heightened sensitivity spiritually, and my body feels great. My joints and muscles are limber and flexible, and my energy level is high.

—MIKE B.

Game Plan

Here is an example of your daily Daniel Diet plan Option Number 1:

- 6:30 A.M.: purified water, 16 ounces

- 8 A.M.: purified water, 16 ounces

- 10 A.M.: purified water, 16 ounces

- 12 P.M.: purified water, 16 ounces

- 12:30 P.M.: grapes (one large bunch), half an avocado, and a handful of raw or soaked almonds and pumpkin seeds

- 2 P.M.: purified water, 16 ounces

- 3:30 P.M.: salad greens, red onion, red peppers, cucumbers, and sprouts topped with a blend of avocado, tomato, red onion, garlic, and lemon juice

- 5 P.M.: purified water, 16 ounces

- 6:30 P.M.: organic fresh strawberries, a half cup of fresh mature coconut or one Thai coconut (you may drink the coconut water), and raw almonds

- 8:00 P.M.: purified water, 16 ounces

You will follow this eating plan on Days 1-9. On Day 10, you should try your best to consume only water and break your Daniel Diet at 5 P.M.

A great way to break the Daniel Diet on the evening of Day 10 is as follows:

- 5 P.M.: drink green vegetable juice (8-16 ounces)

- 5:20 P.M.: consume green salad with organic veggies

- 5:45 P.M.: consume steamed or baked wild fish such as salmon

- 8 P.M.: drink a smoothie

SMOOTHIE RECIPE

8 oz. plain Amasai, yogurt (goat or sheep milk), or kefir (goat or sheep milk)	vanilla extract, to taste (alcohol extract, not glycerin)
2 raw eggs (organic pasture-raised), optional	1 tablespoon extra-virgin coconut oil
1 fresh banana	1 tablespoon raw almond butter (optional)
½ avocado	1 tablespoon cacao powder (optional)
1 tablespoon raw unheated honey	3 tablespoons Terrain Omega or milled sprouted seeds

There's another way you can follow the ten-day Daniel Diet that's super convenient, healthy, and delicious. Beyond Organic has created EA Pulse, which are enzyme-activated organic superfood meals that will power your Daniel Diet. These include raw, sprouted organic fruits, vegetables, nuts, and seeds, and fermented living herbs.

Loaded with antioxidants, fiber, vitamins, minerals, omega-3 fats, probiotics, and enzymes from over thirty superfoods, each EA Pulse blend may be one of the most nutrient-dense meals you've ever consumed. We combine EA Pulse with Terrain Tonic 10, a botanically infused structured water containing ten treasured botanicals that were widely consumed in the days of Daniel and considered as or more valuable than precious metals.

For about the same price the average American spends on food per day, you can have all of your Daniel Diet foods and beverages shipped directly to your door. For more information on the Daniel Diet 10-Day Transformation Pack, visit www.LiveBeyondOrganic.com.

Here is an example of your daily Daniel Diet plan that is Option Number 2:

Option Number 2

- 6:30 A.M.: drink one bottle (16 ounces) of Terrain Tonic 10 (botanically infused structured water)

- 8 A.M.: drink one bottle (16 ounces) of Terrain Tonic 10 (botanically infused structured water)

- 10 A.M.: drink one bottle (16 ounces) of Terrain Tonic 10 (botanically infused structured water)

- 12:30 P.M.: one bag of EA Pulse Antioxidant Fruits (see ingredient list below)

- 2 P.M.: drink one bottle (16 ounces) of Terrain Tonic 10 (botanically infused structured water)

- 3:30 P.M.: consume one bag of EA Pulse Super Veggies (see ingredient list below)

- 4:30 P.M.: drink one bottle (16 ounces) of Terrain Tonic 10 (botanically infused structured water)

- 6 P.M.: drink one bottle (16 ounces) of Terrain Tonic 10 (botanically infused structured water)

- 6:30 P.M.: consume one bag of EA Pulse Omega Fruits (see ingredient list below)

- 8:00 P.M.: drink one bottle (16 ounces) of Terrain Tonic 10 (botanically infused structured water)

You will follow this eating plan on Days 1-9. On Day 10, you should try your best to consume six bottles Terrain Tonic 10 and break your Daniel Diet partial fast at 5 P.M.

A great way to break the Daniel Diet on the evening of Day 10 is as follows. Note that many of the foods and beverages listed below are available at www.LiveBeyondOrganic.com.

- 5 P.M.: drink 8-16 ounces of SueroViv (green is best)

- 5:20 P.M.: consume a green salad with organic veggies, Beyond Organic Greenfed Cheese, and EA Live Seven Seed Crackers

- 5:45 P.M.: consume a Beyond Organic Green-Finished Ranch Roast, sautéed veggies with sweet potato or quinoa

- 8 P.M.: drink an EA Live Smoothie (which will be like a thick pudding)

EA LIVE SMOOTHIE RECIPE

8 oz. plain Amasai	1 tablespoon raw, unheated honey
2 raw eggs (organic pasture-r	vanilla extract to taste (alcohol
1 fresh banana	extract, not glycerin)
½ avocado	1 tablespoon extra-virgin coconut oil
3 tablespoons Terrain Omega or Eaised),	1 tablespoon raw almond butter (optional)
optional A Live Sprouted Seven Blend	1 tablespoon raw cacao powder (optional)

If you're not up for a smoothie, try EA Live Granola Sweet Greens with plain Amasai.

EA Pulse Ingredients

EA Pulse Antioxidant Fruits

Sprouted Seed Clusters (Sunflower Seed,* Coconut (flakes),* Flaxseed,* Chia Seed,* Hemp Seed,* Pumpkin Seed,* Sesame Seed,* Banana,* Date,* Fig,* Mulberry,* Black Sesame Seed*), Superfruit Blend (Goji,* Strawberry,* Raspberry,* Blackberry,* Pomegranate,* Raisin,* Cherry,* Currant,* Cranberry* (sweetened w/Apple Juice), Acai,* Noni,* Mangosteen,* Plum,* Red Apple,* Pink Grapefruit*), Sprouted Nut Blend (Pecan,* Almond,* Cashew,* Walnut*), Terrain Living Herbal Infusion (Fermented Ginger,* Fermented Echinacea,* Fermented Lavender,* Fermented Milk Thistle,* Fermented Cinnamon,* Fermented Rooibos,* and Fermented Ginseng* in a base of live probiotics and enzymes)

EA Pulse Omega Fruits

Sprouted Seed Clusters (Sunflower Seed,* Coconut (flakes),* Flaxseed,* Chia Seed,* Hemp Seed,* Pumpkin Seed,* Sesame Seed,* Banana,* Date,* Fig,* Mulberry,* Black Sesame Seed*), Superfruit Blend (Pineapple,* Mango,* Golden Raisin,* Wild Mountain Apricot,* Peach,* Sea Buckthorn,* Green Apple,* Yellow Grapefruit,* Lemon,* Lime,* Orange,* Tangerine,* Papaya,* Kiwi,* Sprouted Nut Blend (Pecan,* Almond,* Cashew* Walnut*), Terrain Living Herbal Infusion (Fermented Ginger,* Fermented Turmeric,* Fermented Star Anise,* Fermented Lemongrass,* Fermented Black Tea,* Fermented Green Tea,* Fermented Holy Basil,* Fermented Oregano, and Fermented Peppermint in a base of live probiotics and enzymes)
*organic

EA Pulse Super Veggies

Sprouted Seed Clusters (Sunflower Seed,* Coconut (flakes),* Flaxseed,* Chia Seed,* Hemp Seed,* Pumpkin Seed,* Sesame Seed,* Onion,* Portabello Mushroom,* Black Sesame Seed*), Super Veggie Blend (Green Pea,* Corn,* Kale,* Green Pepper,* Green Onion,* Broccoli,* Celery,* Collard,* Green Cabbage,* Green Bean,* Cucumber,* Spinach,* Zucchini,* Lettuce,* Brussels Sprouts,* Asparagus,* Purple Onion,* Purple Cabbage,* Beetroot*), Yellow Squash,* Carrot,* Red Pepper,* Tomato,* Butternut Squash,* Yellow Pepper,* Pumpkin,* Sweet Potato,* Radish*), Sprouted Nut Blend (Pecan,* Almond,* Cashew,* Walnut*), Terrain Living Herbal Infusion (Fermented Garlic,* Fermented Turmeric,* Fermented Star Anise,* Fermented Lemongrass,* Fermented Cinnamon,* Fermented Rooibos,* Fermented Ginseng,* Fermented Black Tea,* Fermented Green Tea,* Fermented Holy Basil,* Fermented Oregano,* Fermented Peppermint,* Fermented Echinacea,* Fermented Lavender,* and Fermented Milk Thistle* in a base of live probiotics and enzymes)

*organic

Please note that I encourage you to refrain from any other foods, beverages, or other commonly consumed items during this ten-day period. This includes but is not limited to coffee, energy drinks, gum, mints, or candy.

If you are on medication and/or under the care of a physician, please consult him or her before beginning this or any diet regimen, *and by no means* should you alter your medication dosage or schedule. Please check the ingredients for each of the EA Pulse products, and do not undertake the 10-Day Daniel Diet if you have known allergies to any of the ingredients.

FLEX OPTIONS FOR THE DANIEL DIET

The Daniel Diet may be the most effective cleanse available, but it can also be extremely challenging. If you find yourself having a difficult time sticking to the program but really want to persevere, we offer the follow flex options.

During the ten-day Daniel Diet, if your appetite and/or food cravings are getting the best of you, or if you find yourself experiencing unbearable detoxification symptoms such as loose bowels, aches, pains, fatigue, etc., we offer five flex meals.

While I believe the best results are achieved by following one of the two Daniel Diet options listed above, you may consume five flex meals during your ten-day Daniel Diet. The Flex Meal should occur in place of your third meal of the day, starting at 6:30 P.M. and ending at 7:30 P.M. It's important to consume the meal within the one-hour allotted time period. Each flex meal can consist of foods from one of three categories with Number 1 being optimal and Number 2 and Number 3 being acceptable alternatives:

1. Consume any raw, fresh organic fruit, vegetable, nut, seed, or raw/cold-pressed vegetable oil (i.e. extra-virgin olive oil)

2. Consume any combination of raw or cooked vegetable, fruit, nut, seed, or gluten-free whole grain (soaked and sprouted is best). Examples are amaranth, quinoa, millet, and buckwheat. You may also consume high mineral sea salt.

3. Consume any biblically correct food from the Recommended Food list (see pages 213-225).

Our goal for you during this ten-day Daniel Diet is to experience wonderful results while feeling your best. Many will have no trouble following one of the two Daniel Diet protocols exactly as written.

Our goal, however, is for everyone to have a successful and comfortable experience while cleansing. Since the concept of fasting is virtually foreign to our modern culture and diet, the flex meals ensure virtually anyone can follow the Daniel Diet to completion.

THE DANIEL DIET DARE

Goals: As a Daniel Diet participant, you're encouraged to set goals (via a 500-word essay) that you'd like to see God accomplish in and through your life in the areas of physical, spiritual, mental, and emotional health.

The Diet: You will be undertaking the Daniel Diet inspired by Daniel 1:12. I was inspired to develop this ten-day diet that I believe accurately represents the diet that Daniel, Hananiah (Shadrach), Misha-el (Meshach), and Azariah (Abednego) consumed—in order to honor God—while they were held in Babylonian captivity.

Prayer: Commit to daily prayer three times per day—both corporately and individually.

Results: You can expect to see fantastic transformation in body, mind, and spirit as God gives you ten times the wisdom, favor, and understanding as husbands, wives, mothers, and fathers, as well as in your leadership, business, job, school, service, athletics, and all areas of your life.

There's another idea I want to share, and I file this under the category of "extra credit." I want to encourage you to "fast" from the popular culture and take a respite from watching TV, surfing for hours on the Internet, and all the "noise" that threatens to sabotage our lives.

You might look at the Daniel Diet as a time to study or practice something you've always wanted to learn. Maybe there's a book on an important topic (such as child-rearing) that you've always wanted to read but never seem to have time for. Perhaps this is your chance to finally listen to those Spanish DVDs from Rosetta Stone that you purchased at the airport but never got around to using. Or maybe this is your time to learn to play a musical instrument.

I hope by now you can see that there are so many compelling reasons to take ten days out of your busy schedule to transform your body, mind, and spirit by following the Daniel Diet.

DANIEL DIET FREQUENCY

If you experience wonderful results from embarking on the Daniel Diet, then I recommend you repeat this ten-day cleanse every three months for a total of four times per year. January, April, July, and October are great times to cleanse with the seasons. A ten-day cleanse can provide amazing benefits for your health and well being, but with the Maker's Diet Revolution, cleansing isn't simply relegated to four times per year.

You may be asking, Now that I've completed the ten-day Daniel Diet, what's next?

Well, I'm glad you asked. In Chapter 2, I'll give you a detailed road map to continue your health transformation through monthly, weekly, and daily cleansing. Before you know it, three months of amazing health will lead right to your next Daniel Diet for ten days!

2

AFTER THE CLEANSE

Now that you've completed the 10-Day Daniel Diet, I want to give you a road-map to continue on the path to cleansing monthly, weekly, and even daily. Best of all, your body will do all the work if you simply remove the interference. The truth is, our bodies were created to cleanse each and every day. All we have to do is get out of the way.

When your body is given the opportunity to repair, restore, and cleanse on a regular basis, you're well on your way to extraordinary health. On the flip side of the coin, when the body *isn't* given the chance to cleanse toxins that build up over time, long-term health challenges can present themselves. I'm convinced that the standard American diet as well as our constant eating are causing our bodies to malfunction. By removing the interference, our bodies can do what they were created to do.

Most natural health disciplines—chiropractic, acupuncture, and mas-sage—are centered around the concept of removing the interference from the body. Chiropractic removes the interference within the spine or nervous sys-tem. Acupuncture removes the interference from what traditional Chinese medicine deems the "energy centers" of the body. Massage removes the inter-ference from the muscles.

If you're consuming unhealthy foods and compounding that error by eat-ing, eating, and eating around the clock, you're interfering with your body's natural cleansing mechanisms. Your body will never have a chance to truly cleanse. You will never reach your health potential. It's a vicious cycle—and a slow, steady downward one at that. You simply can't change the trajectory of your health if you don't cleanse.

Here's an example of what I mean. On our Beyond Organic farms in Missouri, it's impossible to build healthy pasture or forage for our animals if the beneficial plants are constantly overrun by weeds that gain a foothold. Livestock need to munch on greens—grasses, herbs, forbs, and legumes—in order to consume the healthiest diet possible.

What happens when nasty weeds infiltrate a field? In conventional agriculture, the answer is to spray with toxic weed-killers, but the good grass and the bad weeds are sprayed alike. Eventually, the weeds build resistance to the chemicals, and the beneficial plants eaten by the animals weaken in their foundation or root system.

In an organic environment, one way to hold the weeds at bay and to give the preferential forage a fighter's chance is to till everything under six inches or so of soil and give the favorable plants a fresh start to out-compete the weeds by destroying their roots. Likewise, the best way to give your body a fresh start is to complete a ten-day quarterly cleanse such as the Daniel Diet and then continue a maintenance cleansing program, if you will, monthly, weekly, and daily.

By *quarterly*, I suggest repeating the Daniel Diet for ten days every three months. I recommend starting the Daniel Diet on a Monday; that way, you're cleansing during only one weekend, which people seem to appreciate.

By *monthly*, I recommend undertaking a three-day cleanse, which can be accomplished in a number of ways. You can consume only water (which, as mentioned earlier, can be very challenging), or you can drink detoxifying beverages such as raw juices. You can also try drinking herbal infusions, but perhaps the most effective three-day cleanse of all is an exclusive diet consisting of a cultured whey beverage known as SueroViv (see sidebar for more information). These three-day cleanses should span from Monday through Wednesday, Tuesday through Thursday, or Wednesday to Friday.

By *weekly*, I'm talking about cleansing for twenty-four to thirty-six hours one day each week. You could start a one-day-a-week fast on Mondays at 6

P.M. after dinner and fast on water, raw juices, or cultured whey beverages such SueroViv or Suero Gold for twenty-four hours until Tuesday night at 6 P.M., at which time you consume an evening meal. Or, you can choose to carry on until Wednesday morning to make it a thirty-six hour fast.

Better yet, make Wednesday your day to cleanse and call it "Cleanse Day Wednesday." During those weeks that you complete a monthly three-day cleanse, you won't need an additional one day cleanse for that week. You can make your monthly three-day cleanse on Tuesday, Wednesday, and Thursday, which would incorporate your "Cleanse Day Wednesday."

During Jesus' time on earth and into the days of the early Church, it's believed that people of faith fasted once or even twice a week for a twenty-four-hour period. If a ten-day Daniel Diet hits the reset button of life, and the monthly three-day cleanse is a nice tune-up, then a one-day-a-week cleanse is a great way to press the pause button before you get back into action. Please note that every month when you do a three-day cleanse, that replaces your one-day cleanse for that week.

By *daily*, I'm referring to a concept or strategy that will be new to many of my readers. In fact, daily cleansing might be the most controversial yet powerful principle in the Maker's Diet Revolution. I confess that this key element was missing in the original *Maker's Diet* book, but I wasn't aware of its biblical and historical significance at the time.

By daily cleansing, do you mean I have to fast every day, Jordan?

Not exactly, but there is a way you can receive many of the benefits of fasting by practicing daily cleansing, which is an important health strategy that I want to share in this chapter. If you can incorporate the notion of shortening the time from when you take your first bite of food in the day to the time when you take your last bite, you can give your body the necessary time it needs to cleanse on a daily basis.

The Three-Day Suero Cleanse

A three-day cleanse once a month is a great way to support detoxification of the colon, liver, kidneys, and lymphatic system. Many health conditions such as occasional fatigue, joint discomfort, digestive issues, hormonal imbalances, and even brain fog can be linked to excessive toxicity.

I've found a secret weapon for a three-day fast that promotes proper hydration and supports healthy intestinal flora. I'm talking about the consumption of cultured whey, a co-product of cheese production that was called "healing water" more than 2,400 years ago by Hippocrates, the father of medicine.

Cultured whey contains H_2O and an ideal balance of sodium and potassium. Sodium is essential because it pumps water and nutrients into your cells. Potassium functions by pumping waste produces out of the cells.

Beyond Organic has created a certified organic, cultured whey beverage containing vitamins, minerals, probiotics, enzymes, organic acids, and an infusion of essential oils. It's called SueroViv, and it's the cornerstone of a three-day cleanse program with three levels: Bronze, Silver, and Gold. Bronze is the entry level for first-time cleansers, and Gold is the advanced level.

During a three-day Suero Cleanse, you do not eat or drink anything other than six bottles of SueroViv each day. SueroViv comes in five flavors: Green, Citrus, Raspberry Lemonade, Orange Cinnamon, and Gold (which is 100 percent organic, cultured whey from exclusively green-fed cattle with nothing added).

For more information, please visit www.LiveBeyondOrganic.com.

WHAT DAILY CLEANSING IS ALL ABOUT

In 1998, I was in my early twenties, just a couple of years removed from my forty-day health transformation in San Diego when I defeated digestive issues that threatened my well-being and even my life.

The consumption of probiotics was a major factor in my health turnaround. When I returned from San Diego, I did extensive research on the topic of probiotics, determined to gain expertise in this emerging area of nutrition.

Slowly but surely, I began to connect with publishers and editors of publications in the natural health field. One of those publishers was Ori Hoffmekler of *Mind & Muscle Power*, a monthly health and fitness publication for exercise enthusiasts and beginner-to-competitive bodybuilders. Hoffmekler asked me to write a series of articles about probiotics for his audience.

Hoffmekler, a former Israeli Special Forces soldier, wrote an ongoing column entitled "The Warrior Diet." He believed that the Roman gladiators and other soldiers of old "under-ate" during the daylight hours mainly out of necessity, but this practice promoted alertness and the generation of energy. Then they ate large amounts of food in the evening. This practice flies in the face of conventional wisdom, which tells us we should eat large meals for breakfast and lighter meals in the evening.

The concept made sense to me. Just a few years earlier when I was a student at Palm Beach Gardens High School, I could remember frequently falling asleep during my first class after lunch. I know I got my worst grades in those afternoon classes and had to serve the most detention periods for bad behavior. Conversely, the classes I had before lunch were when I excelled at school. The best grades. The best note-taking. And the best behavior.

It was Ori Hoffmekler who introduced me to the concept of "intermittent fasting" or daily cleansing, which is a pattern of eating that alternates between periods of fasting or under-eating and building or overeating. The basis behind the idea of daily cleansing is that there is a ratio between cleansing and building (eating). To determine your ratio, you compare the amount of time you cleanse over a twenty-four hour period to the amount of time from when you eat your first bite of food to your last bite.

I believe the ideal cleansing to eating ratio is somewhere between a 2:1 and 4:1 ratio. This effectively means you're cleansing for at least 16 hours a day and eating for no longer than eight hours (which is how you get the 2:1 ratio). If you can cleanse for a longer time and shorten the time from your first meal to your last, you improve your ratio.

In today's culture, the 2:1 ratio of cleansing to building is usually reversed. I believe this is one of the major reasons why Americans are such an unhealthy people.

Most Americans wake up at 6 A.M. to get ready for work and/or get the kids off to school. At 6:30, they sit down for a bowl of cereal and a cup of coffee. Then it's a mid-morning snack (bagel, doughnut), followed by lunch (sandwich, burger and fries), a cookie in the afternoon, a meat-and-potatoes dinner at 6 P.M., a bowl of ice cream at 9 P.M., and maybe a "midnight" snack from the cookie jar.

I'm exaggerating a bit, but not by much! What I'm trying to illustrate is that many millions of Americans are eating from roughly 7 o'clock in the morning to 11 o'clock at night, which means there are eight hours of cleansing and

16 hours of "building" or eating. Under such a scenario, you have a ratio of cleansing to building of 1:2.

I believe one of the best ways to improve your health, increase your energy, and support detoxification is to increase your daily cleansing time, thus improving your cleansing-to-building ratio. I'm encouraging you to reverse that ratio to at least 2:1—or better. That would mean cleansing in the morning (consuming only water, herbal infusions, raw juices, or cultured whey beverages) and making your first meal of the day at noontime or later. You would eat another small meal or healthy snack at 3:30 and then finish your day with a large dinner at 6 P.M.

With this schedule, you would be eating from roughly 12 noon or even 1 P.M. to somewhere between 6 and 8 P.M., a period of six to eight hours, which would give you a ratio of between 3:1 (18 hours of cleansing and 6 hours of building) to 2:1 (16 hours of cleansing versus eight hours of building).

The reason I'm making a big deal about this ratio is because I'm convinced that the amounts and types of foods that we eat as well as *how long* we eat each day are causing our bodies to malfunction, age prematurely, and pack on the unwanted pounds. I believe if we can shorten the time from when we take the first bite of solid or high-calorie food to the last—even if we ate the same exact food in the same amount during those hours—we would lose weight and feel better.

Here's an example to illustrate how our constant eating can even impact our immune system function. When you eat a meal, a phenomenon called digestive leukocytosis takes place. This means there is an increase in the number of leukocytes, a type of white blood cell, in the bloodstream. When you eat typical foods found in the American diet that are loaded with toxic chemicals and allergens, your leukocytes go on heightened alert and increase in numbers because they feel compelled to mount a defense.

Leukocytes are known as the knights in shining armor—the protectors of our body. One hour after a meal, these defenders go after the things you ate as if they were invaders. Even if you consumed a meal containing healthy organic foods, these white cells are compelled to check things out. That's all for the good, but this process leaves your body vulnerable to an attack elsewhere from germs and toxins. When white blood cells can't keep up, a number of health issues arise.

By following a regimen of daily cleansing, you give your body *more time* to deal with toxins lurking in the body instead of having to answer a three-alarm call in the digestive tract when everything comes down the hatch. Your body knows how to take care of itself if you simply remove the interference. Its job is made easier by daily cleansing and proactively shortening the amount of time from the first meal of the day to the last.

When you follow the Maker's Diet Revolution nutrition plan, you're doing exactly the opposite of what most people do. You'll be cleansing for sixteen to eighteen hours a day and eating or building only six to eight hours a day. I'm not saying that you can't consume anything but water before noon or after six o'clock. You can certainly consume live cleansing beverages. Veggie juices are great. Cultured whey beverages such as SueroViv are extremely beneficial. Unsweetened or lightly sweetened organic tea or coffee is okay. Water infused with liquid herbs can be wonderful as well. But once you start consuming foods—even healthy ones—that starts the clock.

I've heard a lot of talk over the years about controlling certain hormones that regulate hunger and fat storage. It's only been in recent years that scientists have discovered how a pair of "hunger hormones" secreted by the body—leptin and ghrelin—reduce or spike hunger pangs. The hormone leptin, which is generated by fat cells, sends crucial signals to the brain's "satiety center" to stop eating when the stomach is full, kind of like a yellow light at an intersection. The trouble is that many with weight problems have conditioned their bodies to ignore the internal cautionary reminder to stop grazing at the buffet table. With each additional bite, they speed past the intersection of appropriate satisfaction, which is the epicurean equivalent of running a red light—and just as dangerous.

For a long time, people have said that the best way to regulate these hormones is by following a low carbohydrate diet—eating a diet that pretty much consists of only protein and veggies. In my experience from talking with thousands who have tried a low-carb diet, they were miserable eating baked chicken and steamed broccoli and little else. Many can't stay on such a restrictive diet for very long. When they binge, they go off the deep end and wolf down delicious carbs—bread, potatoes, rice, breakfast cereals, ice cream, and a thousand different desserts.

I'm someone who doesn't enjoy a low-carb diet. I can stick with it, but I know that you can receive the same hormonal control by eating a healthy balance of protein, carbohydrates, and fats in a tighter time window. This is yet another reason to be intentional about how long you eat during each twenty-four hour period.

Here's the best news of all: when you practice daily cleansing, you don't have to practice portion control like you do with so many other diets. Your body will control how much you eat and even tell you when enough is enough. You'll feel full and stop eating. You'll begin to crave what you need instead of what you want—perhaps for the very first time.

That's just one of the amazing benefits of following a daily cleansing program.

GOING BACK TO BIBLICAL TIMES

I wanted to see if there was any biblical relevance to this concept of daily cleansing. After all, I knew people didn't eat three square meals a day in the Bible. That's just common sense.

After Jesus learned that his cousin John the Baptist had been martyred, Scripture tells us that He left in a boat to a remote area to be alone. But the crowds heard where he was headed and followed on foot from many towns. They didn't pass any McDonald's drive-thrus on the way—although, on my last trip to Israel, there was a Mickey D's pretty close to the Jordan River.

When Jesus saw the great multitude, He was moved with compassion and healed their sick. Then it was getting late in the day—dinner time—and the disciples told Jesus to send the multitudes away so that they could go into the villages and buy themselves some food.

But Jesus said to them, "They do not need to go away. You give them something to eat."

I'm willing to surmise that most of that crowd hadn't eaten that day. I bet there were more than a few who traveled from towns that were a one- or two-day trip by foot. They probably hadn't packed much if any food with them. Their arms were full carrying a mat to sleep on and a coat to keep warm at night. Backpacks had yet to be invented.

It wasn't uncommon for people in biblical times to skip a meal or two or even three. It was customary among the ancient Hebrews, as well as their contemporaries in the Middle East, to eat only one or two meals a day. The "morning morsel" or "early snack," as it's called in the Talmud—perhaps olives in oil or melted butter with a small piece of crusty bread—was their customary way to "break their fast."

Eating a big meal in the morning was a matter of grave reproach in that culture. Ecclesiastes 10:16-17 says, "Woe to the land whose king was a ser-vant and whose princes feast in the morning. Blessed is the land whose king is of noble birth and whose princes eat at a proper time" (NIV).

A proper time. When would that be?

It wasn't in the morning. When the sun came up, that was the time to tend to your flocks, clean out the stalls, milk the cows, and do your work with perhaps a little something in your stomach. This way of thinking is just the opposite of what you hear today about breakfast being the "most important meal of the day."

Guess who started promoting the idea that breakfast is the most import-ant meal of the day? The cereal makers. When I was a kid, I used to watch Bill Cosby do his little picture pages, and you'd see these public service announcements about breakfast being the most important meal of the day, and then you'd see who sponsored the show. Invariably, it was a big cereal company.

The first meal of the day in biblical times was taken at or just after noon-time—the hottest part of the day when it was also a smart idea to take a rest from labor. It's a tradition that carried over to the days when the United States was an agrarian society up until the start of the 20th century. When field hands came in at noontime and sat around the dining room table, they were presented with their first substantial meal of the day. Think about it: why did farm families call the noon meal "dinner" and the evening meal "supper"—and still do today?

The answer is that the second and main meal of the day in Jesus' time was called supper. Luke says, "Then He said to him, 'A certain man gave a great supper and invited many, and sent his servant at supper time...'" (Luke 14:16-17)

Supper wasn't late in those days. Once it got dark, it got a lot harder to prepare food in the tent or the cave home they were dwelling in. There wasn't a whole lot of light at night.

There weren't a whole lot of fat people back in those times, either. You walked everywhere and performed manual labor for the most part. The mentions of fat people in the Bible are few. The Book of Judges recounts how left-handed Ehud used a double-edged sword to assassinate an evil Moabite king named Eglon, who was described as a "very fat man."

When Eli—"an old man and overweight"—was told that the Ark of the Covenant was taken by the Philistines, he fell backward off his chair and broke his neck and died.

Even though you can go to the Louvre Museum in Paris and see hundreds of paintings with fat angels, young men from biblical times looked like Michelangelo's statue of David—lean and muscular. They were fit because they likely had a narrower time of eating and practiced daily cleansing, whether they knew it or not.

Here's how I put these principles into practice. When I get up in the morning, I start with a 16-ounce glass of pure water along with a supplement of cleansing minerals. An hour or two later, I consume another 16-ounce glass of water with fermented liquid herbs mixed in. An hour or two after that, I may have a cultured whey beverage such as SueroViv.

I know what you may be thinking: *Jordan, how can I not eat a regular breakfast in the morning? What if I have an important meeting? How will I function, stay alert? I can't just drink green juice or cultured whey in the morning. I'm going to be weak and sick.*

You may feel lethargic the first couple of days after you change things around, but soon, very soon, you'll experience more energy and mental clarity. You'll be sharp when participating in your meetings or taking care of the kids. You'll find that you won't be hungry early in the morning because your body knows it should still be cleansing. What will happen is that noontime or later will become your new breakfast and you really will be "breaking your fast" when you consume your meal.

And now with your new daily cleansing routine, you can still say that breakfast is the most important meal of the day, but it's best eaten after noon.

Between noontime and early evening often as late as 5 P.M., I may have a fresh veggie juice followed by some raw cultured veggies. To start dinner, I'll consume a green salad with as many colors as I can: green lettuce, tomatoes, cucumbers, celery, red onions, cabbage, sprouts, red and yellow peppers, and carrots. I'll usually have a dressing that includes extra virgin olive oil and either apple cider vinegar or fermented liquid herbs and a dash of my favorite seasoning Herbamare.

My main entrée will be either wild-caught fish, pastured poultry, or Beyond Organic green-finished beef. I'll have sautéed or steamed veggies on the side, and if I'm going to have something starchy, I'll have a sweet potato or quinoa. (As I write these words tonight, I had my wife Nicki's delicious chili made with Beyond Organic Cheddar Sausage.)

That's my main meal of the day. Two or three hours later, I'll make a smoothie with a Beyond Organic cultured dairy beverage known as Amasai, some pastured eggs, raw honey, banana, avocado, extra virgin coconut oil, raw almond butter, cacao powder, vanilla extract, and a sprouted, fermented organic chia seed and herbal infusion we call Terrain Omega. Or maybe I'll have a serving of sprouted granola with Amasai or green-fed Really Raw cheese with fresh or dried fruit. I've been known to make delicious home-made ice cream from time to time as well.

I know something else you may be thinking: *Jordan, how can you eat that much at one time and not gain weight?*

All I can say is that I've been following this daily cleansing regimen for some time, and it seems like the more I eat during that tight time frame, the more fat I burn and the better I feel the next day.

Let me reiterate this point: I believe so strongly in daily cleansing that if you were to eat the exact same foods in the exact same proportions but during a shorter time window, you would in fact lose weight and feel better. Of course, when you consume the healthiest foods and beverages available, the beneficial results can be exponential.

In fact, if you make a commitment to follow a quarterly, monthly, weekly, and daily cleansing regimen, I wager to say that you'll experience a health transformation before you know it.

3

THE STRUCTURE OF WATER

Since Daniel beseeched Ashpenaz, the head of palace personnel, to "give us pulse to eat, and water to drink," you can see why water is a pretty large component of your health and certainly a key contributor to the efficacy of the Daniel Diet.

When it comes to cleansing, water is the river that hydrates the cardiovascular system, keeps the engine of digestion running smoothly, and lowers body temperature in stifling heat. Water plays a significant role in good health because of the way it revs up your metabolism and irrigates cells so that they can more efficiently process what you eat and drink. When your body's cells are well-hydrated, you accelerate the liver's ability to remove waste and help your kidneys flush out toxins.

Daniel and his cohorts were likely not aware that water regulates body temperature, carries nutrients and oxygen to the cells, makes up 92 percent of their blood plasma, cushion joints, or protect organs and tissues, but they understood that water was necessary to maintain energy, strength, and endurance.

As with many things in life, there's water and then there's *water*. In my experience, the key characteristic of water is its *structure*. What does that mean?

Many people are unaware that water has a unique molecular structure. Japanese researcher Masaru Emoto, author of the fascinating book, *The True Power of Water*, studied the distinctive scientific properties of water by taking water samples from around the world, slowly freezing them, and then photographing them with a high-powered microscope. What he saw was that each water crystal was unique, just as no two snowflakes are alike. But something greater caught Emoto's eye: clean, pristine water created beautifully formed geometrical crystals, while the crystals from dirty, polluted water were either distorted or randomly formed.

In other words, water has much more "structure" to it than anyone ever thought possible and responds to outside forces and agents. The small size of water molecules contradicts the complexity of its actions. When water is in its liquid crystalline form, the molecules move together, much like a school of fish swimming in unison.

Researcher Clayton M. Nolte, who's made it his life mission to study the properties of water, said that structured water is water in its natural form. "If you take a gallon or ten gallons of water and pour it in a mountain stream at the top of the mountain and then collect it at the bottom, the water is structured. Structured water is free of negative energy. It has a balanced pH."

Twenty-five years ago, French scientist Jacques Benveniste rocked the scientific world when he published a research paper in the highly respected journal *Nature* stating that pure water has "memory" of its origin as well as memory of what it's gone through up to present time. In his research, Benveniste started with a substance that caused an allergic reaction. He kept diluting the substance until there was nothing left except for water. That pure water still managed to trigger an allergic reaction when added to living cells. This is very similar to the principles of homeopathic medicine.

Take a Sip of Terrain Tonic 10

Beyond Organic has produced a botanically and structured infused water beverage known as Terrain Tonic 10, which we offer as part of the Daniel Diet 10-Day Transformation Pack. Infused with ten organic fermented botanicals, Terrain Tonic 10 is the perfect beverage to consume during a cleanse or daily as a tonic beverage.

Visit www.LiveBeyondOrganic.com for more information.

Peer review of Benveniste's claims could not be independently replicated in the lab, and it turned out that Benveniste was misled by flawed experiments. One thing scientists agree on, though, is that water can have a different structure under some circumstances because water molecules bond to each other in different ways, forming dif-

Drink Plenty of Water

If you're unable to drink structured water, you can find naturally structured water in the form of natural spring water. At the very minimum, any water you drink must be filtered.

Spring water occurs when water flows to the surface of the earth from underground without man's intervention. When you consider all the water on earth, including the mighty oceans and seas that cover 71 percent of our planet, only 2.7 percent is fresh water, and just a fraction of that amount comes purified by the hydrogeologic formations under the earth. Called "living water" by many health experts, spring waters can range from those high in mineral content to those with lower amounts of solids.

Drinking municipal tap water just doesn't cut it these days. Tap water is routinely treated with chemical agents such as chlorine, chloramines, and fluoride to "scrub" the water—which introduces environmental toxins *and* changes its structure. That's double trouble for water.

The same goes for water marketed as "mineral water." Sure, minerals are great, but the minerals you find in water are generally in a form unusable in the body because when water runs over rocks, the rock sheds minerals, which become part of the water. The liver has to work harder to deal with minerals and trace elements such as zinc, magnesium, and iron from water. These minerals are more bioavailable when they come from foods, so I don't agree that water with a high amount of minerals or solids is the best source for drinking.

Distilled water is a type of water that has its impurities removed through steam distillation, a process that involves boiling the water and condensing the steam into a clean container. This is meant to replicate the process in nature where water turns to steam and rises and condenses in clouds and then rains down to earth as essentially distilled water.

I keep coming back, though, to structured water as the healthiest way to go. Dr. Emoto is convinced that water changes its quality according to the "information" it takes in. In his research, Dr. Emoto exposed water to different types of music—classical Bach, Japanese folk music, and heavy metal riffs—to see what would happen to the composition. Distilled water exposed to classical music took the shape of delicate, symmetrical crystalline shapes. Water samples bombarded with heavy metal chords and a big drumbeat did not form crystals at all but displayed chaotic, fragmented structures.

Some of you are nodding your heads and saying, *I could have told you that would happen.* Based on this and other water research as well as my belief that various frequencies can have a major impact on the structure of water, we play worship music and healing Scriptures at the source of our water used in our beverages and in our dairy parlor where the cows are milked.

The best news of all is that I think our employees who milk the cows have more Bible verses memorized than just about anyone. I think our cows must know quite a few Scriptures by heart as well. Just don't ask them to quote any.

ferent geometrical structures—like the ones that Dr. Emoto viewed with microscopic photography.

Another researcher, Dr. Gerald Pollack, a professor of bioengineering at the University of Washington, studied water's structure and discovered that much of the water in the human body is in a liquid crystalline/structured state. This allows the tissues of the body to work more cooperatively.

Proponents of structured water often stray into New Age terms, declaring that structured water has "life force energy" and a "vortex phenomenon." Putting that aside, there are some scientific insights into structured water that can't be overlooked or denied. Logic should tell us that we should never drink water that has been recycled, polluted at one time, or was former waste-water, if at all possible. Water changes properties when man starts messing with it or polluting it, and that's something we can all agree on.

I've tested structured water both personally and put it to use on our Beyond Organic farms in southern Missouri. My goal was to create a healthy forage base by more effectively growing the desired plants. A key to the growth of healthy plants is properly hydrating the soil and the root system. One of the main benefits of structured water is that the water actually becomes "wetter."

Scientifically, what is happening to the water is a lowering of surface tension, allowing the water to better penetrate the soil and even the root structure of the plants. We have installed multiple structured water units on our farms to be used in irrigation of our pastures and to provide drinking water for our cattle. While we can't prove this scientifically, we, along with several other progressive farmers, can attest to improved pastures, healthier cows, and even an increase in milk production.

You can purchase structured water units that look very much like water filters that you place between the water line coming out of your wall and your kitchen sink, refrigerator, and shower or you can install whole house units.

BE INTENTIONAL ABOUT WHAT YOU DRINK

When you join the Maker's Diet Revolution, you may want to replace your beverage of choice with structured water or other cleansing beverages such as

Drink Up

How much water should you drink?

Probably a lot more than you're drinking now. Perhaps you noticed in the Daniel Diet plan outlined in Chapter 1 that I recommend drinking four 16-ounce bottles of purified water *before* consuming your first meal of the day at 2 p.m. Then the rest of the day, I recommend another three to four additional bottles.

I understand that is quite a bit of water during a ten-day cleanse. However, for the average person on the average day, I operate under the rule of thumb that you should drink one half-ounce of water for every pound of body weight.

Since I started the Daniel Diet, my weight has been hovering around 185 pounds, which means I should drink 92.5 ounces of water or other cleansing beverages per day, which amounts to almost six 16-ounce bottles. I know that's a lot of water—considerably more than a half-gallon—but if you're interested in transforming your health, hydration is a key piece of the puzzle. Exercising will increase your need for fluids, so monitor accordingly.

There's one more reason why I recommend drinking so much water. Drinking water throughout the morning will take the edge off any hunger pangs before your first meal in the early afternoon.

So drink early and drink often.

fresh juices or cultured whey beverages.

I hope that you've kicked the habit of drinking sodas and diet soft drinks, which are terribly unhealthy to consume. Many are sweetened with high fructose corn syrup or non-nutritive chemical sweeteners, which can be devastating to your health and can even become addictive.

It may take some willpower to retrain your taste buds to accept the taste of water, raw veggie juice, fermented herbs, teas, and cultured whey beverages, but once you do, your body will begin to crave the fluid replacement it needs to fuel the trillions of cells that make up your healthy body.

4

THE POWER OF PULSE

This will probably be no surprise to you, but I'm going against the grain again in this chapter.

Grains make up the major ingredients in breads, cereals, cakes, and a zillion other processed foods these days. Grains are a staple of the standard American diet due to the energy they convey in the form of carbohydrates.

Wheat, rye, and barley have been around ever since humankind shifted from a nomadic lifestyle to staying in one place and planting crops nearby. Somewhere along the line, ancient people discovered that grinding threshed grains into a powder (flour), adding a leavening agent such as yeast, and baking the dough in wood-fired ovens made delicious bread and added a foundational element to their diets. Bread is often used as a synonym for "food" in the Bible, and Jesus even called Himself the "bread of life" in John 6:35.

So how could Jesus compare Himself to bread if bread is considered unhealthy by many today?

Answer: because bread in Jesus' time was vastly different from today's commercially made breads, buns, muffins, and rolls, which use hybridized, chemical-laden, refined white flour as their main ingredient.

With the introduction of machinery during the Industrial Age, man found a way to take something healthy—our grains—and turn them into something totally unhealthy by stripping away the God-given vitamins, minerals, and fiber content during the refining process.

Every day, more than 200 million Americans consume food products made of refined, bleached, and unbleached wheat flour. They'll have:

- a breakfast consisting of a bowl of sugar-coated cereal or make a quick stop for a Danish during the morning commute

- a mid-morning snack of perhaps a glazed donut or toasted bagel

- a lunch consisting of a turkey sandwich made from "enriched" white bread or a hamburger on a sesame seed bun

- a dinner consisting of pizza or some type of pasta dish

- a dessert of apple pie with a crust made from refined flour, or perhaps a pastry or cupcake

The list is endless. I'm not even including all the chips and crackers that people love to snack on before and after meals. Those are made from refined grains or starches as well.

Then there's the issue of gluten, the sticky protein found in wheat, rye, and barley. Gluten is presenting health challenges for millions of people these days. All you have to do is open a restaurant menu and find the section offering gluten-free options. To this growing customer base of people who suffer from gluten intolerance, the topic of grains has become a big deal in the last decade.

So if you're thinking that I'm going to come down hard against grains, here's where I go against the conventional wisdom. I'm actually in favor of consuming grains, as long as they are grown organically *and* are consumed in a soaked, sprouted, or fermented/sour leavened form. I'm especially fond of ancient *non*-gluten grains such as amaranth, millet, quinoa, and buckwheat, as well as sprouted nuts and seeds.

A big component of the Daniel Diet is seeds, which are a main ingredient in our EA Pulse blends. What I want all of us to do is eat the very best grains and seeds available. To accomplish that goal, I've come up with a hierarchy of grains that goes like this:

🖋 At the bottom of this totem pole are the grains common in the American diet—mainly wheat that's been processed and refined into white bleached and unbleached flour and is used to make every processed food known to man.

🖋 Next up are whole grains, which are a step above processed grains but not much because the wheat and other cereal grains come from conventionally-treated soils where pesticides, herbicides, fungicides, and chemical fertilizers are routinely used.

🖋 Organic whole grains are better than conventionally-grown whole grains for reasons you might surmise. In their natural state growing in organic soil, whole grains are the seed of the plant. A grain seed is made up of three key edible parts—the bran, the germ, and the endosperm—and is surrounded by a husk that protects the kernel from assault by sunlight, pests, water, and disease.

While the protective components of whole grains keep pests from destroying the seeds, they contain nutrient and enzyme inhibitors and thus can be difficult to digest and can even rob nutrients from the human body.

🖋 Sprouted or sour-leavened organic whole grains, flours, cereals, and pastas come next. *Sprouting*, also known as germination, is a time when a seed comes to life and the nutrient potential trapped within the seed is unleashed. Sprouting is a great way to increase the digestibility of whole grains, seeds, nuts, and legumes while maintaining their nutrient density.

When seeds are allowed to germinate or sprout, this increases the enzymatic activity and inactivates substances called enzyme inhibitors. Enzymes are essential for digestion, cellular energy, tissue and organ repair, and brain activity and should not be inhibited.

Enzymes, the driving forces behind virtually every biochemical reaction that occurs in the human body, are tiny proteins that help turn food into energy and unlock this energy for use in the body. Without enzymes, life would slow to a standstill because chemical reactions inside our bodies wouldn't happen.

Sour-leavened is a term that refers to a process in which grains and seeds are mixed with a starter culture, and a "pre-digestion" process ensues that allows the nutrients to be more easily assimilated and absorbed by the body. Sour leavening uses a sourdough starter made from beneficial yeasts and bacteria, or it can come from wild yeasts in the air. You can find instructions for making your own sourdough culture or purchase yeast-free, whole grain sourdough bread from your health food store or grocery.

Coming in at Number 2 on the totem pole are non-gluten grains such as amaranth, millet, quinoa, and buckwheat. These non-gluten grains are personal favorites of mine, and I try to include one of them in my meals when I'm looking to add a healthy source of carbohydrates to my plate. These four grains are actually classified as seeds and contain a higher percentage of proteins and less starch than other grains. They are much less likely to cause allergies and are easily digested by many who cannot tolerate gluten-containing grains.

At the top of the totem pole are seeds, preferably sprouted or germinated seeds that will give you everything that grains provide—vitamin E, plenty of B vitamins, essential fatty acids, fiber, and more—and are free of gluten, higher in protein, and lower in carbs than grains. They also contain much less starch.

Sprouted seeds are rich in digestible energy, bioavailable vitamins, minerals, amino acids, proteins, beneficial enzymes, and phytochemicals—necessary elements for a germinating plant to grow. Sprouting increases the content of plant enzymes, raises the quality of protein, gives us essential fatty acids, and provides for the chelation of minerals. Sprouting accomplishes a veritable pre-digestion of grains, which is great for our bodies.

Dr. Edward Howell, a leading physician and biochemist of the 20th century and author of *Enzymes for Health and Longevity*, stated that germination increases enzyme activity by as much as six times. Soaking the seeds allows proteases within to neutralize the enzyme inhibitors and to release the enzymes from bondage.

The process of germination not only increases vitamin C but also favorably alters the composition and nutritional profile of the seed. Sprouting increases vitamin B content, especially B2, B5, and B6. Meanwhile, carotene dramatically increases—sometimes *eightfold*.

Even more importantly, sprouting neutralizes enzyme inhibitors present in all seeds such as phytic acid, a substance found in the bran of all grains, which blocks the absorption of calcium, magnesium, iron, and zinc.

These inhibitors can also neutralize our own precious enzymes in the digestive tract. Additionally, complex sugars responsible for intestinal gas are broken down during sprouting. Sprouting also inactivates aflatoxins, which are potent carcinogens found in grains, seeds, and legumes. Finally, numerous enzymes that help digestion are created and liberated during the germination process.

THE SEVEN SEEDS

I recommend consuming the following seven organic seeds in their sprouted, enzyme-activated form each and every day. They're wonderful in recipes, trail mixes, cereals, nut and seed butters, cookies, crackers, bars, and, when in a powder form, great in smoothies.

Chia seeds are packed full of fiber and are high in healthy fats such as monounsaturated fats and omega-3 fatty acids. Indeed, chia's fiber-rich seeds have the highest percentage of omega-3s of any plant, including flaxseeds. You'll also find plenty of calcium, phosphorus, manganese, potassium, and antioxidants in chia seeds, which help support healthy blood sugar levels and cardiovascular health and provide fiber for satiety and healthy weight management.

Flaxseeds are an excellent source of soluble and insoluble fiber as well as omega-3 fatty acids. You'll find eight vitamins, four macro-minerals, four trace minerals, and ten amino acids in flaxseeds.

Sesame seeds have been prized by ancient cultures because of their belief that they promote energy and longevity. Sesame seeds contain the antioxidants sesamin, sesamolin, and sesamol as well as calcium, magnesium, zinc, iron, B1, phosphorus, and fiber. The lignans in sesame seeds support healthy cholesterol levels, blood pressure levels, and liver health. Women of ancient Babylon ate sesame seeds to promote youth and beauty, while Roman soldiers consumed sesame seeds for strength and energy.

Black sesame seeds have been used in traditional Chinese medicine and Ayurvedic medicine to address the underlying physical disturbances that lead to aging and premature gray hair. Black sesame seeds, which can be used as a flavoring agent in many dishes, support the health of the bowels and promote the health of the liver and kidneys.

Hemp seeds are rich in omega-3 and omega-6 fatty acids. They are also an excellent source of gamma linoleic acid (GLA) and contain the highest percentage of protein of any seed or grain. No other single plant source has the essential amino acids in such an easily digestible form.

Sunflower seeds, which promote healthy digestion and weight management, are packed with vitamins, including vitamin B1 and B5, vitamin E and folate, and provide important minerals such as copper, magnesium, selenium, and phosphorous. Sunflower seeds are nature's gift from the beautiful sunflower and its rays of petals branching out from a bright yellow, seed-studded center.

There are folklore stories about Russian soldiers who were given around a cup of sunflower seeds each day as their food allotment, and they were able to live for days and weeks on nothing but sunflower seeds. In modern times, major league baseball players—especially those seeking to break a chewing tobacco habit—dig out handfuls of sunflower seeds from their back pockets, popping them into their mouths and spitting the shells into the breeze.

Pumpkin seeds are usually thrown away after carving a pumpkin, but these flat, green, and crunchy seeds are highly nutritious and flavorful. Pumpkin seeds are especially rich in omega-3, omega-6, and omega-9 fatty acids as well as beta-sitosterol, which supports the good HDL cholesterol in the blood. The consumption of these seeds support healthy prostate function in addition to providing carotenoids, iron, zinc, manganese, magnesium, phosphorus, copper, and potassium.

So go against the grain and begin consuming any of these seeds in their sprouted form today.

INTRODUCING EA LIVE

EA Live from Beyond Organic is a revolutionary technique based on ancient wisdom.

Each organic nut and seed undergoes an exclusive enzymatic activation process utilizing structured, energized water and an ancient symbiotic culture to increase nutrition and digestibility and to decrease enzyme inhibitors and anti-nutrients. The delicate enzymes, vitamins, and minerals are preserved within each ingredient through our raw food air-drying system.

Enzyme-activated foods are rich in digestible energy, bioavailable vitamins, minerals, amino acids, proteins, beneficial enzymes and phytochemicals. They increase plant enzyme content and protein quality while conveying essential fatty acids, chelation of minerals, and vitamin content. On the other hand, it also reduces anti-nutritional factors such as phytic acid.

Enzyme activation accomplishes a veritable pre-digestion of nuts and seeds. Phytic acid, which blocks the absorption of calcium and magnesium, is largely decomposed, while certain sugars are made more digestible.

At Beyond Organic, we have created a complete line of delicious and nutritious foods and snacks using our Sprouted Seven Seed Blend, including seasoned nuts and seeds, trail mixes, cereals, cookies, crackers, bars, and even a gluten-free, organic, sprouted baking mix for use in cooking, baking, and smoothies. The foods and snacks are designed to add easily digestible nutrients and beneficial fiber to your everyday diet.

Visit www.LiveBeyondOrganic.com for more information.

5

THE RAW REVOLUTION

I'm sure by now you've realized that one of the principles behind the 10-Day Daniel Diet is the consumption of fresh fruits, vegetables, nuts, and seeds—or three bags of our specially formulated EA Pulse daily—all in their raw or live form.

I'm well aware that other diets based on the book of Daniel present you with a meal plan comprised of chickpea and lentil soup and heaping helpings of steaming pinto beans—cooked foods. So why is my Daniel Diet focused on consuming raw live foods? Was that intentional?

The answer is *yes* because I've become a staunch believer in the power of raw nutrients in their unheated, untreated, and unadulterated form. Since the writing of *The Maker's Diet,* I've become an even bigger believer in the power of raw foods, which are loaded with live nutrients that include vitamins, minerals, probiotics, enzymes, and undenatured amino acids.

Raw foods are called "live" foods because they are consumed in their original, unheated—meaning uncooked—state, which makes them raw and alive. Examples of raw foods include fruits, vegetables, nuts, seeds, sprouts, grains, and legumes in sprouted form, fresh veggie or fresh fruit juices, and even animal foods such as dairy, eggs, and meats, which can be consumed raw.

Even though many people don't think about eating raw food as much as they should, many of us intuitively understand that raw foods are the best sources of every known nutrient available. Let me explain why I feel this way.

I've presented thousands of seminars on the subject of health and nutrition at churches, health food stores, and wellness expositions over the years. Sometimes when I step before an audience, I pose this simple question:

If someone offered you an apple from a tree or a small jar of applesauce made from the very same apple, which would you choose?

You should see the eyes light up and the hands go in the air. Everyone is eager to tell me, "The apple!"

And they would be correct because a raw apple, picked from a tree at harvest time, will always be more nutritious and more alive than applesauce, which is a purée of cooked or baked apples.

When an apple is peeled and cooked, you lose all of the enzymes and probiotics contained in and on the apple, and many of the vitamins are partially or completely destroyed, including half of the fruit's vitamin C content. Even though the very same apple was used to make the sauce, it doesn't take a rocket scientist to figure out that a fresh raw apple trumps processed applesauce every time.

That's why the Daniel Diet eating plan is centered around consuming raw live foods, which are—in my opinion and with few exceptions—the healthiest forms of food available. During the first nine days of the Daniel Diet, you'll greatly benefit from consuming a diet of raw foods in the form of fruits, veggies, and nuts, or consuming the combination of over ninety raw superfoods that we call EA Pulse. No matter which route you take, you'll be receiving the best form of vitamins, minerals, and bioactive compounds available.

Of course, I understand that Daniel, along with Hananiah, Misha-el, and Azariah, may not have exclusively eaten raw pulse when they were sitting at the king's table while their Babylonian counterparts wolfed down "delicacies" supplied by the palace kitchen. I wouldn't be surprised, though, if they consumed plenty of raw fruits, veggies, nuts, and seeds as part of their ten-day eating regimen.

As someone who's been a huge proponent of the raw food movement and pioneered the creation of the very first raw food multivitamins known as The Vitamin Code®, green foods known as Perfect Food®, probiotics known as RAW Probiotics®, enzymes known as RAW Enzymes®, and even the first raw, organic, and plant-based protein powder and meal replacement known as RAW Protein® and RAW Meal®, I understand very well the power of consuming raw nutrients. When it came to formulating EA Pulse, I knew from the beginning that we had to use raw whole food ingredients and bioactive compounds in their most usable, easy-to-digest form. That meant using ingredients that were unheated, untreated, and unadulterated.

The idea of consuming raw foods isn't a new concept. Adam and Eve, we're told in the Bible's first book of Genesis, subsisted on raw fruits, vegetables, seeds, and nuts in the Garden of Eden. Certainly throughout biblical times people ate much of their food raw and made raw nuts and seeds cornerstones of their diet, especially during the winter months when fresh fruit and vegetables weren't readily available.

Fast forward to present times, when our high-tech world has figured out how to take fresh fruits, farm-grown vegetables, and raw nuts and seeds and process these nutrient-dense gifts from God into manufactured, microwave-friendly, and mass-produced foods that are anything but healthy for us.

We need to swing the pendulum back to eating raw live foods as quickly as possible.

RAW FOOD AND ENZYMES

One of the biggest benefits of a raw food is the abundance of enzymes it contains. Enzymes are small bioactive proteins that act as catalysts, meaning they speed up chemical reactions in the body. Enzymes, as I explained in the last chapter, help the body turn food into energy and then unlock this energy for use in the body.

The enzymes present in raw foods play a vital role in our health because if you're not supplying your body with the enzymes it needs to break down the foods you eat and produce biochemical reactions, then the body will deplete the stores of enzymes already present, placing a burden on your enzyme-producing organs such as the pancreas. While the body's digestive system produces a substantial number of different enzymes, the body needs specific enzymes that can only be obtained directly from raw foods in the diet.

To help you better understand enzymes, below are the three types of enzymes your body utilizes:

- *Metabolic enzymes* are produced by the pancreas and perform a wide variety of functions. Breathing, eating, sleeping, digestion, absorption of nutrients, muscular movement, growth, blood circulation, immune system function, and sensory perception all are dependent on metabolic enzymes.

- *Digestive enzymes* are utilized in the digestive tract, where they aid in the digestion, absorption, and utilization of food. Digestive enzymes are produced by the pancreas in response to eating cooked food. When we eat raw foods, the pancreas doesn't need to produce as many enzymes or potentially none at all.

- *Food enzymes* are found only in raw unheated foods and help initiate the process of digestion in the mouth and stomach. So while our digestive organs produce enzymes internally, the rest must come from live foods such as fresh fruits and vegetables, raw sprouted seeds and grains, and raw unpasteurized dairy products, to name a few.

Food enzymes are vital to the body because they can help pre-digest the food before it reaches the small intestine, thereby reducing the need for the pancreas to produce more digestive enzymes. This is another reason the Daniel Diet consists of raw live foods.

I don't believe, however, that you need to consume an entirely raw diet all the time, although there are periods when it makes sense—such as when you cleanse each quarter, month, week, and even at times during each day.

In addition, I believe that most people should consume more raw live foods in their diet because too many meals are consumed away from home in restaurants, which serve mainly cooked and processed food. Everyone agrees that consuming more fresh greens, vegetables, and fruits is an excellent way to reach optimal health, but few see that through. You can be part of the solution.

WHAT FOODS SHOULD BE EATEN COOKED?

As much as I like raw foods and what they can do for the body, I recommend that a few certain foods be cooked. If you're going to consume grains, I believe the cooking process makes them more digestible.

Likewise, when certain fibrous vegetables such as cauliflower and broccoli are cooked, the heating process softens the fiber and makes them more digestible in my opinion. Same with legumes and beans, which should be ideally soaked overnight and then baked or boiled. Nuts and seeds, when consumed raw, may also cause some digestive complaints, which is why I recommend soaking and sprouting.

THE TOP ENZYME-RICH RAW FOODS

I have some personal favorites when it comes to consuming raw foods. Here are a few:

- **Avocados,** with their creamy rich texture, provide protein, healthy monounsaturated fats, and enzymes galore, especially lipase, the fat-digesting enzyme. If my salad doesn't have avocado, I feel like something is missing.

- **Bananas** are another enzyme-rich food, but note of caution: the more bananas ripen, the more enzymes that are utilized in the process. Try to eat bananas before they are overripe.

- **Pineapple** is the main source of bromelain, a protein-digesting enzyme that has been used for centuries to support healthy inflammation. The less ripe the pineapple, the more enzymes.

- **Papaya**, a fruit native to Central America and tropical latitudes, contains the protein-digesting enzyme papain, which has a mild and soothing effect on the stomach. When isolated, papain is used as a meat tenderizer because of the way it breaks down proteins.

- **Mangos** originated in Southeast Asia and are grown in Mexico, Haiti, the Caribbean, and South America. You'll find enzymes in mangos that stimulate the metabolism and detoxify the intestines. Again, the less ripe the fruit, the greater the enzyme content.

- **Alfalfa sprouts** contain enzymes such as lipase to break down fat; amylase and sucrase, which break down carbohydrates and convert them into easy-to-digest sugars; pectinase to digest starches; and protase to digest proteins. Sprouts such as alfalfa also contain antioxidant enzymes such as SOD (super oxide dismutase) and catalase.

- **Raw sauerkraut** is a fermented veggie blend that is consumed as a healthful food in various cultures around the world, but here in this country, most commercially-available sauerkraut is processed with heat and made with vinegar, which eliminates the naturally occurring enzymes beneficial to the digestive tract. When sauerkraut or cultured veggies are made simply with probiotic cultures, salt (optional), and good old-fashioned time, they are amazing foods to support digestive and immune system function.

Consuming more raw live foods is a critical part of the Maker's Diet Revolution eating plan. By placing an emphasis on the consumption of nutrient-dense, enzyme- and probiotic-rich raw foods, you'll eliminate cravings for many unhealthy—and even *addictive*—foods in your daily diet.

You may experience an increase in food cravings, have mild headaches, or even undergo changes in bowel habits as you integrate more raw, nutrient-dense, and high-fiber foods into your diet, but those will be minor bumps in the road and long forgotten after you experience a transformation in mind, body, and spirit during your Maker's Diet Revolution.

6

FAT AND FIBER: FAITHFUL FRIENDS

Since much of the Maker's Diet Revolution is centered upon cleansing and reducing excess pounds, I thought this would be a good place to talk about two important factors that will keep those pounds off and increase the amount of toxins leaving your body.

When it comes to managing weight, supporting healthy blood sugar levels, and effectively promoting detoxification of the body, we have two dietary allies, or as I call them, *faithful friends*—fat and fiber.

The former is a macronutrient, and the latter is a component of the carbohydrate portion of plant foods that the body can't digest or absorb. Although dietary fiber is not digestible, it is very important for digestion, elimination, and overall health. Fiber keeps the digestive tract healthy, particularly the colon, pulls out excess hormones and toxins from the body, provides a food source for the good probiotic bacteria, and promotes healthy cholesterol levels.

I'll be getting into more detail about fat and fiber soon, but let me set the stage a bit by reminding you that one of the biggest essentials for maintaining a healthy weight comes from balancing appetite-regulating hormones such as leptin and ghrelin, the "hunger hormones" that can reduce or spike hunger. But there's another hormone that we have to pay attention to, and that's insulin.

Insulin is a hormone produced by the pancreas to deal with blood sugar known as glucose that comes into the body via our diet. When you consume a high-sugar food, even a piece of fruit, the pancreas secretes insulin with orders to either shuttle the sugar into the cells for energy or store it as excess fat.

I'll give you one guess where that excess fat is stored.

Sugars, as well as starches, are carbohydrates. It's generally accepted that the more refined the carbohydrates—think about the ingredients in most any processed food you find on a supermarket shelf—the harder the pancreas has to work to produce insulin to deal with that sugar, either as energy for the cells or as excess fat.

Carbohydrates come mainly in two forms—monosaccharides and disaccharides. (There is a third form called polysaccharides, but for the sake of argument, disaccharides and polysaccharides have two or more sugar molecules, so for this discussion we'll consider them essentially one and the same.)

Monosaccharides are comprised of a single sugar. Most fruits, vegetables, natural cheeses, cultured dairy products, raw honey—and nuts and seeds—contain carbohydrates that are mainly in the form of monosaccharides. The gastrointestinal tract finds monosaccharide foods easier to digest because these single-molecule carbohydrates can be absorbed through the lining of the small intestine without having to be digested or broken down first.

Disaccharides are composed of *two* molecules of single sugars that are linked together. Examples of disaccharide-rich foods are grains, potatoes, table sugar (sucrose), and corn. The most common American dietary sources of disaccharides are foods containing refined white or brown sugar or processed grains such as boxed cereal, bread, bagels, dinner rolls, and blueberry muffins.

Disaccharides are *much* more difficult to digest. When unabsorbed carbohydrates remain in the large intestine undigested, they feed harmful bacteria and upset the balance of the intestinal flora—prompting digestive problems to strike. Eating an abundance of disaccharide-containing foods can also result in malabsorption in the gastrointestinal tract, which means that food travels too rapidly through the digestive tract, leading to nutrient deficiencies and digestive issues.

When you consume foods high in sugars or starches—even those commonly believed to be healthy, such as carrot juice or grapes—with a fat or a fiber, or both, something good happens in the body. Fat and fiber slow the absorption of the sugars and, therefore, cause a decreased insulin response, which promotes balanced energy levels and mood and leads to a longer period of post-meal fullness.

In recent years, there has been much discussion about this topic based on the development of the glycemic index, which measures how foods affect blood sugar levels and, specifically, how quickly the carbohydrates in foods are broken down into sugars. Here's some good news: when you add a fat or fiber to food with a high glycemic index—a food whose sugars are quickly absorbed by the body, such as juice or a piece of fruit—the glycemic index is lowered.

I've noticed that some weight-loss companies are basing their entire message on a "low glycemic" diet. Based on the science of the glycemic index, the way you manipulate the glycemic index is by increasing fiber and fat in food.

One of the secrets of success for the Daniel Diet is the consumption of meals that are balanced with healthy fats and fiber. If you look at the balance of protein, carbohydrate, fat, and fiber in the foods recommended on the 10-Day Daniel Diet such as seeds, nuts, avocados, coconut, and the EA Pulse blends, you'll find that these foods are slowly absorbed and the sugars are very slowly released into the body, which makes them ideal for supporting healthy blood sugar levels.

About Those Carbs...

I have a saying that I've repeated for years: *Don't eat carbs naked.*

What I mean is that it's not a good idea to eat carbohydrates—starches and sugars—naked, or by themselves. You should be consuming fat and fiber along with your carbs because they slow the absorption of sugar into the bloodstream, which keeps insulin levels in check.

Those insulin levels are something you want to pay attention to, especially if you're the parent of young children. I know it's popular to hand your kids a boxed juice, but even if they're drinking a healthy, natural juice not made from concentrate, that juice quickly turns to sugar in the bloodstream, which ramps up insulin production. This could set your youngster down a path that leads to insulin insensitivity, which could lead to pre-diabetes. Likewise, constant and excessive insulin production is one of the culprits of obesity and diabetes.

The next time your child reaches for a glass of healthy juice, be sure to have him or her eat a handful of sprouted seeds or nuts—good sources of both fat and fiber.

That's why fats and fiber are your allies. You're not going to get fat eating foods with good fats; you gain weight by consuming high-carbohydrate foods loaded with sugars and starches that quickly release into the bloodstream as glucose and cause a spike in insulin, triggering fat storage. You certainly don't gain weight by eating high-fiber foods such as celery, cucumber, soaked and sprouted nuts and seeds, and berries.

I encourage you to add healthy fat to your diet. I want you to add fiber to your diet. And I want you do be intentional about adding *both* in combination whenever possible.

A LOOK AT FAT

I'm amazed at how many people still think that fat is bad for you. They've been told by "health experts" for decades that fat makes you fat, which reveals a huge misunderstanding in the way the body works. It's eating foods with excess carbohydrates, especially processed foods, that kicks up the insulin levels and cause the body to store the surplus around your midsection.

Fats are vital factors in the diet, necessary for normal growth and proper function of the brain and nervous system. The right fats protect our bodies' organs and systems and help us maintain optimum energy levels. Good fats are found in a wide range of foods, including those of animal origin such as pasture-raised beef, lamb, poultry, eggs, fish such as wild-caught salmon, and organic dairy products such as Amasai, butter, and cheese.

When I formulated the Daniel Diet, I wanted to find healthy foods and meals that contain both fat *and* fiber in the right ratio. Topping my list, once again, is my faithful friend, the humble avocado.

Avocados may have a little more fat than fiber, but there's a reason why avocados are a part of my daily diet and have been for years. Avocados are high in healthy monosaturated fats as well as important vitamins and minerals.

Fiber? The creamy flesh contains 10 to 13 grams of fiber (for a medium-sized avocado), right up there with broccoli, cauliflower, and artichokes—foods that are best consumed cooked, as compared to avocados, which are almost always eaten raw.

There's nothing better than several thick slices of a ripe avocado garnishing a salad, which is why I made sure that avocados were part of the Daniel Diet (for those choosing to prepare their own foods). The creamy flesh is not only delicious, but it's really a "two-fer" when it comes to giving your body the fat and fiber it needs during the 10-Day Daniel Diet and every day on the Maker's Diet Revolution eating plan.

Another food that can bat from both sides of the dietary plate is coconut. The coconut meat scraped from the inside of its shell contains copious amounts of fiber and powerful medium-chain fatty acids. Coconut can do a clean-up number on stored toxins, leaving your digestive tract spic 'n' span.

The benefits of coconuts have been known for centuries. Early Spanish explorers, who called the hairy nut a *coco* (meaning "monkey face") because of the three indentations or "eyes" on the shell, soon discovered that coconuts provided a nutritious source of water (or coconut juice, as some call it), milk, meat, and oil. Many island civilizations in the Caribbean and South Pacific depend upon the coconut as a staple in their diet.

Coconut is best eaten fresh or dried. The biggest problem with eating fresh coconut meat is that coconuts have a very short shelf life, and getting to the meat is not for the faint of heart. If you do it yourself, you'll need leather gloves, an ice pick, a hammer, and curved-ended oyster knife. I've split dozens of mature coconuts over the years, and I can assure you there is a learning curve. Young coconuts and Thai coconuts can be good for you, but there's not a lot of fiber in the meat, which has a jelly-like appearance. Best to choose mature coconuts for your fat and fiber needs.

For those who prefer to leave the ice pick and hammering to someone else, dried coconut is available in many forms. As long as the dried coconut is certified organic and hasn't been heated above 114 degrees Fahrenheit, you have a great source of raw fat and fiber. If you're wondering about extra-virgin coconut oil, which I've touted in all of my books, that's a great source of fat but you're missing the fiber.

After avocado and coconut, the other high fat and fiber foods that I want to encourage you to eat are the "Seven Seeds" that I introduced in Chapter

4, "The Power of Pulse." I'm referring to chia seeds, flaxseeds, sesame seeds, black sesame seeds, hemp seeds, pumpkin seeds, and sunflower seeds.

Soaking seeds in water neutralizes the enzyme inhibitors present in all seeds and encourages the production of beneficial enzymes. They're a *lot* easier to digest when soaked. The amount of time you soak depends on the size and the nature of the seeds.

A good way to soak/sprout nuts and seeds at home is to soak the seeds overnight in water, drain and rinse, and then put them in a dehydrator to give them some crispness. It does take a little planning, but once you soak your chia seeds or flaxseeds the first time or two, you'll get the hang of things.

Soaking your seeds for one to three days gives them a chance to sprout, which increases the nutritional profile of your seeds—and nuts. Sprouting increases vitamin B content and neutralizes phytic acid, which is a substance that inhibits the absorption of calcium, magnesium, iron, copper, and zinc. Numerous digestive enzymes are produced during the germination process.

You might find it more convenient to consume our Beyond Organic EA Live foods and snacks, which use an ancient symbiotic culture—in the soaking and sprouting process—to create these foods high in healthy fat and fiber. The enzyme-activated process can be described as "super sprouting" and unlocks the nutrition inside the hulls of seeds and nuts in ways that will make these ordinary foods into superfoods.

Visit www.LiveBeyondOrganic.com for more information.

7

EAT YOUR COLORS

When I began to put together the finer points of the Daniel Diet, I was on a quest to make it the most balanced and effective whole food eating plan possible. One way to accomplish this goal was to ensure that each Daniel dieter consumed fruits and veggies with a wide array of colors.

Why are pigments in fruits and vegetables important other than giving us a visual feast for the eyes that makes each morsel of food so appetizing?

The short answer: highly pigmented fruits and veggies are chock-full of phytochemicals, which offer antioxidant protection as well as other health benefits. The idea of "eating your colors" is one I've long championed as being critical to good health because of the broad array of vitamins, minerals, and antioxidants found in pigmented fruits and vegetables. You'll never go wrong consuming raw fruits and vegetables exhibiting the radiating colors of God's rainbow.

Pigments with health-promoting properties color every fruit and vegetable on display at your local farm, health food store, or green market. Green vegetables owe their pigment to chlorophyll. Tomatoes and watermelon are red because of a carotenoid antioxidant known as lycopene. Blueberries—a favorite in the Rubin household—are colored by the phytochemical anthocyanin, which is also found in blue, black, and purple fruits such as açai berries, blackberries, and dark plums.

Lycopene and anthocyanins act as powerful antioxidants, which are nature's way of fighting off potentially dangerous molecules—known as free radicals—in the body. Antioxidants are compounds that preserve and protect cells and other components of the body from free radical damage.

Under the microscope, free radicals are oxygen molecules with a single electron, but these unstable molecules love to attack the healthy cells of the body. Thankfully, there's an antidote to the voracious electron appetite of free radicals, and that's antioxidants. Since antioxidants do a great job of neutralizing free radicals, you better have a steady supply of antioxidants coming into the body—through fresh foods such as fruits and vegetables—because the body cannot produce antioxidants on its own. If you don't consume a wide variety of fruits and veggies, free radicals will gain the upper hand, and that's not good for your long-term health.

Here's an analogy to describe what antioxidants do to those free radicals roaming around your body with mayhem on their minds. I want you to think of a fire, burning and crackling inside a fireplace. Sparks come off the fire, which is why prudent folks place a screen in front of the fireplace—to catch those sparks so they don't burn the house down.

In a similar way, there's a raging fire inside your body, setting off sparks, or free radicals, but those sparks won't harm you if you put a screen of antioxidants in front of them—yet another reason to eat your fruits and vegetables, especially in a raw form.

Unfortunately, the standard American diet is woefully deficient in antioxidants. You can see it in the colors on people's plates, and those colors are uniformly brown and monochromatic beige. Meals at diners and fast-food restaurants—burgers and buns, fried chicken, breaded fish, mashed potatoes with gravy, grits, and corn are mainly lighter and darker hues of beige and brown with a dash of pale yellow.

What's missing, of course, are the colorful veggies and fruits that not only make meals more visually appealing but also make them much healthier. Many of the vivid colors in fruits and vegetables—the reds, greens, oranges, purples, and yellows—come from phytochemicals such as anthocyanins, phenolics, lutein, indoles, flavonoids, and carotenoids such as lycopene. These beneficial compounds help the body maintain good memory function, cardiovascular health, and a healthy weight.

Pigments with health-promoting properties color every fruit and vegetable. Let's break it down by the color:

- Purple/blue: blueberries, blackberries, purple grapes, plums, prunes, raisins, currants, elderberry, black mission figs, eggplant, beets, and purple cabbage.

- Yellow/orange: oranges, peaches, nectarines, papayas, pineapples, grapefruit, tangerines, mangoes, lemons, apricots, sweet potatoes, cantaloupe, carrots, yellow squash, yellow and orange peppers, pumpkin, and corn.

- Green: salad greens, kiwi, broccoli, avocados, Brussels sprouts, chives, green onions, parsley, celery, asparagus, cilantro, green beans, spinach, peppers, Swiss chard, and kale.

- Red: tomatoes, raspberries, apples, strawberries, pomegranates, cherries, red peppers, radishes, red onion, and watermelon.

- White: bananas, pears, dates, peaches, coconut, potatoes, Turkish figs, jicama, cauliflower, garlic, ginger, mushrooms, onions, leeks, shallots, artichokes, and bamboo shoots.

These colors have been associated with excellent health benefits.

Blue/purple fruits and vegetables support urinary tract health, promote memory function, and support cellular and brain health.

Yellow/orange fruits and vegetables do the heavy lifting against free radicals that roam around your body, looking for cells they can damage. Yellow/orange fruits and vegetables support cardiovascular health and healthy inflammation levels.

Green fruits and vegetables support the body's detoxification efforts and promote a healthy heart.

Red fruits and vegetables support healthy inflammation levels as well as cardiovascular health.

White fruits and vegetables nurture intestinal function and support healthy blood sugar levels and a healthy immune system.

I've compiled a list of twenty of the top commonly available high antioxidant fruits and veggies, based on ORAC (Oxygen Radical Absorbance Capacity), which measures the total antioxidant power of foods. Next to each fruit and vegetable, I've included the ORAC units per 100 grams, or about three and a half ounces, as measured in a study conducted by researchers at Tufts University in Boston.

Leading nutritional researchers believe that you should strive to consume approximately 10,000 ORAC units daily to promote health, wellness, and longevity. When you include the following foods in your diet, meeting that goal should be a cinch:

FRUITS

- blueberries (2400)

- blackberries (2036)

- strawberries (1540)

- raspberries (1220)

- plums (949)

- oranges (750)

- red grapes (739)

- cherries (670)

- kiwi fruit (602)

- pink grapefruit (483)

VEGETABLES

- kale (1770)

- spinach (1260)

- Brussels sprouts (980)

- alfalfa sprouts (930)

- broccoli (890)

- beets (840)

- red bell pepper (710)

- onion (450)

- corn (400)

- eggplant (390)

As you can see, blueberries top the leader board when it comes to antioxidant power, another reason why blueberries should become as popular in your home as they are in mine. If you can find ways to include kale and spinach, which are slightly bitter-tasting greens, into your salads and juices, then you'll really give your body a huge antioxidant boost.

Antioxidants are often overlooked, which they shouldn't be, especially because they come in such beautiful, vibrant colors. So open your eyes and your body to the wonderful health benefits of antioxidants and eat your colors today.

THE COLORS IN EA PULSE

When you're on the Daniel Diet and following my ten-day meal plan, you'll be having a fruit meal in the early afternoon—purple grapes, red watermelon, orange cantaloupe—as well as a light green avocado. The main meal of the day is a salad with multiple varieties of lettuce, red onion, red and yellow peppers, purple cabbage, orange carrots, green and white cucumbers, and white sprouts topped with a blend of light green avocado and red tomatoes. There are a lot of great colors in that salad.

If you're consuming EA Pulse on your Daniel Diet, you'll quickly notice the colors in the bite-size fruits and veggies contained in each blend. Here are some of the "colors" to look for in each of the EA Pulse blends:

EA PULSE ANTIOXIDANT FRUITS

- Red: cherry, red grapefruit, currant, cranberry, red apple, strawberry, raspberry, goji berry, cinnamon, rooibos, and ginseng

- Blue/purple: açai, plum, raisins, blackberry, mangosteen, echinacea, lavender, milk thistle

- White: noni, coconut, Turkish fig, mulberry, dates, banana, and ginger

EA PULSE OMEGA FRUITS

- Yellow/orange: pineapple, peach, golden raisins, orange, lemon, yellow grapefruit, mango, tangerine, papaya, sea buckthorn, wild mountain apricot, turmeric, and star anise

- Green: kiwi, lime, green apple, lemongrass, green tea, holy basil, oregano, and peppermint

- White: coconut, Turkish fig, mulberry, date, banana, and ginger

EA PULSE SUPER VEGGIES

- Red: radish, red pepper, tomato, cinnamon, rooibos, and ginseng

- Yellow/orange: butternut squash, yellow pepper, sweet corn, pumpkin, sweet potato, carrot, turmeric, and star anise

- Green: green pea, kale, green onion, broccoli, celery, collard, green cabbage, green bean, cucumber, spinach, zucchini, lettuce, Brussels sprouts, asparagus, green tea, holy basil, oregano, and peppermint

- Blue/purple: purple onion, purple cabbage, beetroot, eggplant, Echinacea, lavender, and milk thistle

- White: coconut, onion, mushroom, and garlic

8

YOUR CLEANSE CALENDAR

I'm a visual person who likes to see things so that I can commit them to memory. Perhaps you're the same way, too, although I understand that there are two other learning styles—auditory (learning by hearing) and kinesthetic (learning by experiencing the topic firsthand).

I want to share with you my three-month Maker's Diet Revolution Cleanse Calendar that will show you how to structure, organize, and plan your 10-Day Daniel Diet and subsequent monthly, weekly, and daily cleansing program.

My first goal for you is that you embark on the Daniel Diet and stick with it for ten days to receive the body, mind, and spiritual transformation that many others have already experienced. If you do nothing else but follow the Daniel Diet just one time, it was worth my writing this book.

But I don't want you to slip back into old habits of unhealthy eating. In order to keep your health moving forward and build upon all the good you've accomplished, I highly suggest you commit to a three-month cleansing program by completing a three-day cleanse each month, a one-day cleanse each week on "cleanse day Wednesday," and daily cleansing by eating within a six- to eight-hour window, taking your first meal sometime between noon and 2 P.M. and finishing up with your last bite by 8 o'clock at night.

Wonder what that looks like? Me, too, which is why I took the liberty of creating a three-month Maker's Diet Revolution calendar for you.

So, do you have any questions? Need a review? Please feel free to return to Chapter 2, "After the Cleanse," to review the timing and the protocol for the

10-Day Daniel Diet, the three-day monthly cleanse, the weekly cleanse for twenty-four to thirty-six hours, and, of course, the daily cleansing regimen.

JUNE

SUN	MON	TUE	WED	THU	FRI	SAT
						1
2	**3** Day 1 of the Daniel Diet	**4** Day 2 of the Daniel Diet	**5** Day 3 of the Daniel Diet	**6** Day 4 of the Daniel Diet	**7** Day 5 of the Daniel Diet	**8** Day 6 of the Daniel Diet
9 Day 7 of the Daniel Diet	**10** Day 8 of the Daniel Diet	**11** Day 9 of the Daniel Diet	**12** Day 10 of the Daniel Diet Fast all day, eat a regular meal at 5 P.M.	**13** Daily Cleanse (eat within a 6-8 hour window)	**14** Daily Cleanse (eat within a 6-8 hour window)	**15** Daily Cleanse (eat within a 6-8 hour window)
16 Daily Cleanse (eat within a 6-8 hour window)	**17** Daily Cleanse (Eat within a 6-8 hour window)	**18** Daily Cleanse (Eat within a 6-8 hour window)	**19** Cleanse Day Wednesday	**20** Daily Cleanse (eat within a 6-8 hour window)	**21** Daily Cleanse (eat within a 6-8 hour window)	**22** Daily Cleanse (eat within a 6-8 hour window)
23 Daily Cleanse (eat within a 6-8 hour window)	**24** Daily Cleanse (eat within a 6-8 hour window)	**25** Three-Day Monthly Cleanse	**26** Three-Day Monthly Cleanse	**27** Three-Day Monthly Cleanse	**28** Daily Cleanse (eat within a 6-8 hour window	**29** Daily Cleanse (eat within a 6-8 hour window
30 Daily Cleanse (eat within a 6-8 hour window)						

JULY

SUN	MON	TUE	WED	THU	FRI	SAT
	1 Daily Cleanse (eat within a 6-8 hour window)	**2** Daily Cleanse (eat within a 6-8 hour window)	**3** Cleanse Day Wednesday	**4** Daily Cleanse (eat within a 6-8 hour window)	**5** Daily Cleanse (eat within a 6-8 hour window)	**6** Daily Cleanse (eat within a 6-8 hour window)
7 Daily Cleanse (eat within a 6-8 hour window)	**8** Daily Cleanse (eat within a 6-8 hour window)	**9** Daily Cleanse (eat within a 6-8 hour window)	**10** Cleanse Day Wednesday	**11** Daily Cleanse (eat within a 6-8 hour window)	**12** Daily Cleanse (eat within a 6-8 hour window)	**13** Daily Cleanse (eat within a 6-8 hour window)
14 Daily Cleanse (eat within a 6-8 hour window)	**15** Daily Cleanse (eat within a 6-8 hour window)	**16** Daily Cleanse (eat within a 6-8 hour window)	**17** Cleanse Day Wednesday	**18** Daily Cleanse (eat within a 6-8 hour window)	**19** Daily Cleanse (eat within a 6-8 hour window)	**20** Three-Day Monthly Cleanse
21 Daily Cleanse (eat within a 6-8 hour window)	**22** Daily Cleanse (eat within a 6-8 hour window)	**23** Three-Day Monthly Cleanse	**24** Three-Day Monthly Cleanse	**25** Three-Day Monthly Cleanse	**26** Daily Cleanse (eat within a 6-8 hour window	**27** Daily Cleanse (eat within a 6-8 hour window
28 Daily Cleanse (eat within a 6-8 hour window)	**29** Daily Cleanse (eat within a 6-8 hour window)	**30** Daily Cleanse (eat within a 6-8 hour window)	**31** Cleanse Day Wednesday			

AUGUST

SUN	MON	TUE	WED	THU	FRI	SAT
				1 Daily Cleanse (eat within a 6-8 hour window)	**2** Daily Cleanse (eat within a 6-8 hour window)	**3** Daily Cleanse (eat within a 6-8 hour window)
4 Daily Cleanse (eat within a 6-8 hour window)	**5** Daily Cleanse (eat within a 6-8 hour window)	**6** Daily Cleanse (eat within a 6-8 hour window)	**7** Cleanse Day Wednesday	**8** Daily Cleanse (eat within a 6-8 hour window)	**9** Daily Cleanse (eat within a 6-8 hour window)	**10** Daily Cleanse (eat within a 6-8 hour window)
11 Daily Cleanse (eat within a 6-8 hour window)	**12** Daily Cleanse (eat within a 6-8 hour window)	**13** Daily Cleanse (eat within a 6-8 hour window)	**14** Cleanse Day Wednesday	**15** Daily Cleanse (eat within a 6-8 hour window)	**16** Daily Cleanse (eat within a 6-8 hour window)	**17** Daily Cleanse (eat within a 6-8 hour window)
18 Daily Cleanse (eat within a 6-8 hour window)	**19** Daily Cleanse (eat within a 6-8 hour window)	**20** Three-Day Monthly Cleanse	**21** Three-Day Monthly Cleanse	**22** Three-Day Monthly Cleanse	**23** Daily Cleanse (eat within a 6-8 hour window)	**24** Daily Cleanse (eat within a 6-8 hour window)
25 Daily Cleanse (eat within a 6-8 hour window	**26** Daily Cleanse (eat within a 6-8 hour window	**27** Daily Cleanse (eat within a 6-8 hour window)	**28** Cleanse Day Wednesday	**29** Daily Cleanse (eat within a 6-8 hour window)	**30** Daily Cleanse (eat within a 6-8 hour window)	**31** Daily Cleanse (eat within a 6-8 hour window)

Part II

BUILDING YOUR BODY

9

TRANSFORM YOUR TERRAIN

Now that you've cleansed, it's time to rebuild.

For those of you who've never accomplished an extended fast before, the 10-Day Daniel Diet may have felt like a significant reboot of the body's operating system. For perhaps the first time in your life, your organs, tissues, bloodstream, lymphatic system, and digestive tract received a long "holiday." You should be feeling an incredible sense of victory, especially after you stepped on a scale and saw in black and white that you lost a considerable amount of weight in ten days. Cleansing your body of toxins and giving your digestive system a prolonged period of down time is an extremely healthy practice.

So what's next?

I've made the case about the importance of continuing to cleanse on a monthly, weekly, and daily basis as a way to maintain the health improvements you've experienced. Now I want to introduce the second phase of the Maker's Diet Revolution, which is *rebuilding and restoring* the body's internal ecosystem.

What I'm talking about is transforming your terrain.

Terrain? Isn't that a geographical term referring the lay of the land?

Yes, but I'm talking about a different type of terrain—the internal environment of the body. A 19th-century French scientist, Claude Bernard, coined the term when he said "the terrain is everything" after hypothesizing that germs alone could not make a healthy person sick because the person's *milieu interieur*—French for internal environment or terrain—was your defense against toxic invaders.

Bernard literally put his theory where his mouth was. The French scientist drank a glass of water infected with cholera, but he didn't get sick! Bernard took the risk, he said, because he knew he was healthy, had a strong immune system, and believed his body would fight off the germs. When a colleague, Louis Pasteur—yes, the Pasteur of pasteurization fame—heard about Bernard's crazy stunt, he called him "lucky."

But think about the millions of doctors, nurses, and health workers who are around sick people all day long, breathing in germs and coming into physical contact with toxins. Yet they often avoid symptoms of ill health. Why does that happen?

It's because the body's terrain was armed with the proper defense mechanisms. Once you train your terrain, yours can be properly equipped as well.

The backstory about the discovery of the body's terrain is an interesting one that I—a health history buff—loved researching.

We start our journey by going back to the period between 1775 and 1875, a century of time marked by the phenomenal changes throughout the Western world as scientific discoveries, labor-saving inventions, and technological innovations opened the door to the Industrial Age. This pivotal era was also marked by social upheaval: the thirteen original American colonies declared their independence from England and formed the United States, followed by the violent French Revolution and its Reign of Terror, which lopped off the heads of the monarchy and noble class and sent shivers through palace walls from London to Vienna.

France fell under the dictatorship of a victorious general, Napoleon Bonaparte, who enacted a uniform and modern administrative system, gave land tenure to the peasant proprietors, and left the bourgeoisie—the upper or merchant class—a political heritage that they claimed during the 19th century.

I relate this history lesson to help you understand why France, from its Napoleonic height in 1812 to its stunning defeat in the Franco-Prussian War of 1870-71, exerted a powerful diplomatic influence in the civilized world, shaped Western thought, and pioneered noteworthy scientific advancements throughout much of the 19th century. "France led Europe in theoretical and industrial chemistry, and her self-sufficiency during the Revolutionary and Napoleonic Wars was in no small part the result of her scientific superiority," wrote author René Dubos.

Many of the scientific discoveries that impact our health today came from the fertile minds of three 19th century French scientists: Louis Pasteur, Claude Bernard, and Antoine Béchamp. It turned out that Pasteur gained immortality while Bernard and Béchamp became historical footnotes, which is a shame. As you'll soon learn, Louis Pasteur, the father of the pasteurization process as well as the antibiotic age, promulgated a huge mistake 150 years ago, and the repercussions are being felt by millions of people today.

PASTEUR'S GERM THEORY

The hospital was the last place you wanted to go when you were sick in the 19th century. You went to the hospital to die, not to be cured. If leeches, bloodletting, torturous surgery without anesthesia, or benign neglect didn't kill you, then infectious germs would hasten your ultimate demise.

Physicians and scientists still had no idea what germs were in the mid-19th century, but they were getting warm. The first breakthrough came from Dr. Ignaz Semmelweis, a Hungarian physician posted at the Vienna General Hospital, site of the world's largest maternity clinic, in the 1850s. Most women still gave birth at home back then, attended by a midwife, but "problem pregnancies" ended up at Vienna General.

The problem was that too many mothers and too many children were leaving in wooden coffins because mortality rates were ten, even twenty times higher inside the maternity ward than at home. No one knew why the mortality rate was so high. Doctors rubbed their bearded chins and blamed poor ventilation or crowded conditions in the maternity ward.

Dr. Semmelweis noticed something about his colleagues at Vienna General: doctors left the dissection room with their hands bloodied from working on cadavers and didn't do much more than give their hands a cursory wipe on a towel before reporting to the delivery room, where they assisted in bringing a newborn into the world. No washing, scrubbing, or rubber gloves in those days.

On a hunch, Dr. Semmelweis established a new policy: from now on, doctors had to scrub their hands in chlorinated water after working on cadavers. (Dr. Joseph Lister of Scotland wouldn't discover how to kill germs with heat and antiseptics for another eighteen years.) Within a month, the mortality rate in the maternity ward dropped sixfold to 2 percent! Dr. Semmelweis wrote a book about his discovery, which was released in 1861, a year before Pasteur and Claude Bernard completed their first pasteurization test—a process that eradicated undesirable microorganisms through heating—on April 20, 1862.

The middle of the 19th century was a time when huge strides were being made in the scientific world. Two scientists—Antoine Béchamp and Robert Koch, a German scientist and physician—were also conducting pioneering experiments in the area of chemistry, particularly in the areas of fermentation, yeast, and the discovery of microscopic organisms called bacteria.

That same year, 1862, Louis Pasteur was working with curved neck flasks that allowed contact with air but inhibited movement of non-gaseous particles. From these experiments, Pasteur demonstrated that microorganisms were present in the air but not created by air, which led him to theorize that:

- Germs, or microbes, caused disease.

- Germs invade the body from the outside.

- Human blood is sterile and can be infected only by outside microbes.

- The shapes and colors of microorganisms are constant.

- Every disease is associated with a particular microorganism.

- Germs should be killed at all costs by chemical drugs.

In other words, since germs cause disease, it was medicine's challenge to find the right drug or vaccine to kill these germs or prevent the nasty bug without killing the patient first. This theory hardened into a scientific dogma that is considered conventional wisdom in the halls of medicine today. Pasteur's so-called "germ theory" is widely hailed as the single most important contribution by the science of microbiology for the general welfare of the world's people. Furthermore, you could say that the paradigm of modern medical treatment was based on Pasteur's germ theory of disease. Diagnose the germ—for example, a bacteria, virus, parasite, or fungi causing the illness—and then prescribe something to destroy it or make the patient feel better.

Claude Bernard, even though he counted Pasteur as a friend, didn't agree with his colleague's germ theory. He believed germs and microorganisms were constantly changing within the body's internal environment—the terrain. Bernard's research convinced him that the body was constantly striving to maintain a stable, well-balanced environment, one that would not be overly affected by outside influences.

Bernard was a quiet soul who never set out to become a doctor or physiologist. Born in 1813 as the son of poor vineyard workers living in Saint-Julien, France, the young Bernard was educated in a simple village school and dreamed of becoming a playwright. He set off for Paris at the age of twenty-one. A well-known critic, Saint-Marc Girardin, gave his writings the once-over and imperiously announced that young Bernard may want to do something else with his life than pen stage plays.

Bernard accepted the critic's rebuke and applied to medical school in Paris. Despite finishing at the bottom of his class, Bernard passed his studies and obtained a medical degree and moved into the research field, where he gravitated toward experiments centering on the digestive process. He read about a U.S. Army surgeon named William Beaumont, who became known as the "father of gastric physiology" after he devoted several years peering into the digestive tract of a patient who was shot in the stomach. Beaumont's patient had survived the shooting, but the hole in his stomach never healed, which allowed the American doctor to observe the digestion process with his very own eyes.

Beaumont performed this research by tying a piece of food to a string and dropping it through the hole in the patient's stomach. Every few hours, the

American physician would slowly reel in the string and observe how well the food had been digested. This novel research led to the important discovery that digestion was a chemical process, not a mechanical one. Stomach acids, or gastric acids, digested foods into nutrients the body could use.

Claude Bernard replicated Beaumont's work by creating artificial fistulas, or openings, in live animals such as horses. What the Frenchman discovered was that the stomach was not the sole digestive organ; much more digestion took place in the small intestine. He also demonstrated the importance of the pancreas, whose secretions of enzymes broke down protein and fat molecules. Bernard also discovered a sugar-like substance in horses' livers, which he named glycogen.

Then Bernard turned his attention to the portion of the nervous system that governed blood circulation and how the red blood cells carry oxygen from the lungs to body tissues. Each of his findings convinced him that the body's *milieu interieur* was continually striving to maintain a stable, well-balanced state. Disease, therefore, was caused by variations in the body's terrain, to which the microbes responded by changing form to survive.

"The living body, though it has need of the surrounding environment, is nevertheless relatively independent of it," he wrote. "This independence, which the organism has of its external environment, derives from the fact that in the living being, the tissues are withdrawn from direct external influences and are protected by a veritable internal *milieu,* which is constituted, in particular, by the fluids circulating in the body."

Bernard's legacy is that germs could not make a person sick unless the person's internal environment—or terrain—was weak.

ANOTHER CONTRARIAN VIEW

Antoine Béchamp, another French scientist who lived during the 19th century, also crossed swords with his colleague Louis Pasteur. Béchamp's theory was that germs were the *consequence* of disease, not the cause.

Béchamp, who lived from 1816-1908, was one of France's most prominent researchers and biologists. He earned degrees in biology, chemistry, physics, pharmacy, and medicine, and he practiced, researched, and taught in all those disciplines—up until the day he died at the age of ninety-one. The reason why you've never heard of Béchamp is because he called Pasteur's theory that nearly all diseases were caused by germs "the greatest scientific silliness of the age."

Béchamp's voice was ignored by the elites guarding the gates of traditional medicine in the latter half of the 19th century. As Pasteur's germ theory gained widespread acceptance in clinics and classrooms, it laid the foundation for modern medicine's view that doctors should diagnose the disease and then write the proper prescription for "treating" the illness.

Today's medicine is practiced that way: you describe your symptoms to the doctor, he or she diagnoses what ails you, and you walk out with a prescription—often for an antibiotic. Béchamp's contrarian view stated that it was not the germ that caused disease but rather the condition in which the bugs lived in the *milieu interieur,* or internal terrain.

Disease happened when an imbalance in the body's terrain allowed the dangerous or pathogenic microbes, including bacteria, to take over. Béchamp insisted that the germ was not the main focus, but rather what should be studied was the body's terrain, where microbes or germs live.

So, to reiterate, we have two completely different viewpoints or worldviews: Pasteur was certain that germs caused disease, while Béchamp argued that an imbalance in your body's internal systems causes or allows germs to flourish in the body.

Here's where their stories get really interesting. There's strong evidence that Louis Pasteur, at the time of his death, recognized that his lifelong preoccupation with his "germ theory" had been misdirected all along. On this deathbed, he reportedly whispered: *Le germe n'est rien; c'est le terrain qui est tout.*

Translation: "The germ is nothing; it's the terrain that's everything."

From all the reading and studying I've done, I agree completely with Béchamp, Bernard, and (arguably) Pasteur's final words—the terrain *is* everything. Health problems come from *inside* the body, not from the outside. Scientists today know that there are microorganisms that cause—or at least contribute—to certain diseases, but I maintain that germs can thrive only in an unhealthy body—just as termites only munch on wooden homes with a weakened structure.

That's why the Maker's Diet Revolution's cleansing and building plan is designed to help you create an impenetrable terrain that will support your overall health. You should be taking intentional steps to make sure that your terrain is as healthy as possible. Doing so will help you defend against the toxic enemies of your health.

One of those important steps is being sure to include fermented foods and beverages and their beneficial compounds—probiotics, enzymes, and, most importantly, organic acids in your diet. I'll be introducing the concept of fermentation in the next chapter.

10

THE SECRET OF SOUR

Cleansing and building are natural dualities when it comes to good health.

Thanks to Antoine Béchamp, you should have an excellent grasp on the importance of building up the body's terrain. Although Béchamp was swept up and dumped into the dustbin of history, we wouldn't know as much today about germs and their causation without his early insights into the germ theory. For example, thanks to Béchamp, we know that taking steps to improve your body's terrain by consuming naturally soured, fermented foods is an excellent way to balance your body.

You may have picked up on the phrase *naturally soured* in connection with fermented foods. I imagine you did so because the word *sour* is not a pretty expression in the English language nor often meant to be something positive or complimentary.

If you hear that someone is a "sour puss" or has a "sour personality," that tells you all you need to know. Another common expression—"That left a sour taste in my mouth"—reveals deep disappointment. Synonyms for sour including the following descriptive terms: unpleasant, nasty, disagreeable, unlikable, undesirable, distasteful, unappetizing, unpalatable, unsavory, offensive, repulsive, repugnant, and disgusting. I'm not trying to pile on, but you get the point.

Sour, when not used to describe one's personality, also describes how a food or beverage tastes to you. Sour is one of the four basic sensations of taste—sweet, sour, salty, and bitter. Actually, there's a fifth taste perceptible to the 10,000 taste buds on your tongue, and it's called umami (pronounced *oo-MAH-mee*), which is a meaty, savory taste popular in Asian cuisine. Here in this country, American palates are acutely aware of two tastes that we like—sweet and salty—and two tastes we'd rather avoid—sour and bitter.

Let's not sugarcoat things (although we do all the time): Americans *love* sweet and salty foods. Breakfast cereal is sweet, mid-morning muffins are sweeter, midday burgers-and-fries leave a salty aftertaste, tortilla chips at snack time are coated with salt, a meat-and-potatoes dinner is a salt fest, but dessert is *always* sweet.

We don't like to stray too far from the sweet-and-salty comfort foods that we were raised on, which is too bad because our national taste for sweet and salty foods has, in my opinion, destroyed the health of Americans. Consuming sweet things only begets cravings for more sweet-tasting foods, and those sugars and empty calories may be the root cause of the obesity epidemic in this country.

We have a salt habit that's hard to shake, too. Like horses that can't stop using a salt lick, American taste buds crave salty snacks such as chips, bacon, and crackers. Canned soups, condiments, sauces, cold cuts, and canned vegetables are also loaded with salt. The current recommendations from U.S. government health officials state that we should consume less than 2.4 grams of sodium per day, or the equivalent of one teaspoon of table salt, but the body has an actual need for one-fifth that amount. Yet Americans consume two to five times more salt than needed to maintain the right balance of fluids in the body, to deliver water and nutrients into the cells, and to help transmit nerve impulses, which is what salt is needed for.

Salt consists of two minerals—sodium (40 percent) and chloride (60 percent)—but it's the sodium in salt that causes so many health concerns today. The excessive consumption of sodium raises blood pressure and has been linked to strokes because when the kidneys can't eliminate enough sodium, the sodium accumulates in the blood. Increased blood volume makes the heart work harder to move blood throughout the cardiovascular system, which increases pressure in the arteries. Next thing you know, your blood pressure numbers are elevated.

When I think about how many millions of Americans habitually munch on sweet and salty foods from the time they wake up until the time they go to bed, I feel my blood pressure rising. That's overstating things, but I will say that I'm disheartened when I think about how sour and bitter foods have been politely sidestepped in this country. You don't see people clamoring for Brussels sprouts or chopped cabbage or the tart and tangy taste of fermented dairy foods—unless their store-bought yogurt has been sweetened with sugary flavors and artificial sweeteners. They prefer something sweet or salty in their mouths at every meal and with every snack.

It's really a shame that many are unwilling to even try sour-tasting foods and beverages, which are known for their cleansing- and digestion-supporting properties, among other health benefits.

There's power in sour, as you'll see in this chapter.

THE HISTORY OF FERMENTATION

Sour or tart-tasting foods have been around since farmers and shepherds learned thousands of years ago that a natural process called *fermentation* could preserve their foods beyond harvest and extend the freshness of their fruits, veggies, and dairy products. In the process, ancient cultures discovered that fermentation improved the vitality of their foods and made them easier to digest as well as more nutritious. In fact, naturally fermented foods have become prized in every civilization known to man.

Since refrigeration hadn't been invented back then—and foods weren't known to have a "shelf life"—people in ancient times didn't have the option of freezing food or storing any foodstuffs inside a fridge. Instead, they learned how to preserve foods through the process of fermentation.

Fermentation, also known as culturing, is the intentional growth of bacteria, yeast, or mold that breaks down substances to their more basic constituents and creates organic acids that act as natural preservatives. This process can be called pre-digestion and preserves foods over longer periods of time and conveys health benefits beneficial to the body.

What happens is that bacteria and yeasts act upon a food to break down its protein into amino acids, fats into fatty acids, and complex sugars into single sugars such as glucose. This is not a destructive process but is known as "nutritional alchemy," because new beneficial compounds are created during fermentation—probiotics, enzymes, antioxidants, and organic acids, all of which support a healthy terrain.

A classic example would be sauerkraut, which contains higher levels of vitamin C and B vitamins than the cabbage that it originally came from, purely due to the fermentation process. If unpasteurized and uncooked—in other words, produced in a raw state—sauerkraut contains live lactobacilli and other beneficial microbes. Natural or traditional fermentation spurs bacterial growth that gobbles up the natural sugars in the food and produces a tart-tasting organic acid known as lactic acid.

Organic acids are natural preservatives that inhibit the proliferation or growth of putrefying bacteria. Starches and sugars in vegetables and fruits are converted into organic acids by many species of friendly bacteria and yeasts. These microbes or germs are everywhere, present on the surface of living things and especially numerous on leaves and roots of plants growing in or near the ground.

The proliferation of probiotics in fermented vegetables enhances their digestibility and increases vitamin levels. These beneficial microorganisms produce numerous helpful enzymes as well as other beneficial compounds. Their main byproducts—organic acids—not only keep vegetables and fruits in a state of preservation but also promote the growth of healthy flora or probiotics throughout the intestinal tract.

In other words, the organic acids produced in fermentation are important for the maintenance of the terrain and the promotion of healthy digestion and elimination. Several beneficial organic acids are produced during natural fermentation that are worth noting—lactic acid, acetic acid, succinic acid, and gluconic acid. Each of these organic acids help support healthy pH balance in the digestive tract, particularly in the colon, which is critical for proper absorption of nutrients and healthy elimination.

These organic acids also act as natural preservatives due to their anti-microbial effects, but none of this science was known by the early practitioners of fermentation, which started long ago with fermenting cabbage into sauerkraut, grape juice into wine, grains and water into beer, various vegetables into relish, and cow, goat, and sheep's milk into a variety of fermented foods such as yogurt, kefir, Amasai, cheese, cottage cheese, and cultured cream.

We don't know when fermentation was first practiced, but we are aware that the Romans learned to ferment cabbage, which is known today as sauerkraut. Eastern Europeans discovered ways to pickle green tomatoes, peppers, and lettuce. The Chinese also fermented cabbage, and Koreans became skilled at preparing *kimchi*, a condiment composed of cabbage with other vegetables, herbs, and spices. And in nearly every culture, milk from cows, goats, and sheep have been used to make fermented foods such as yogurt, Amasai, cheese, and kefir for centuries.

Kefir, a fermented beverage that's gaining in popularity, is getting much easier to find these days in ready-to-drink quart bottles at natural food stores. This tart-tasting, thick beverage contains naturally occurring bacteria and yeasts that work synergistically to provide superior health benefits. Kefir—best consumed from goat's milk—is also a great base ingredient to build smoothies around. Just add eight ounces of kefir into a blender, an assortment of frozen berries or fruits, a spoonful of raw honey, and you're well on the way to churning up a delicious, satisfying smoothie.

Just as kefir has made a splash in the last ten or fifteen years, much like yogurt did in the 1960s, I believe the next craze in cultured beverages is a newly introduced product into the United States called Amasai. This African-inspired cultured dairy beverage, which tastes like a combination of yogurt and kefir, is made from specially selected cattle similar to the recipe used by the famed Maasai tribe of Kenya. With the taste, nutrient density, and acceptability of a cow's milk product coupled with the tolerability of a sheep or goat milk product, I believe Amasai has all the earmarks of a sensational cultured beverage.

Fermented beverages such as Amasai and SueroViv—the cultured whey beverage that I introduced in Chapter 2—have become personal favorites of mine. The vitamins, minerals, probiotics, enzymes, and organic acids provide the body with the tools it needs to build a healthy terrain.

While we're talking about fermented beverages, there are two more that I want to call to your attention. The first is kombucha or Tibetan tea. Kombucha (pronounced *kom-BOO-cha*) is a fermented beverage made from black tea and a fungus culture. Thought to be Himalayan in origin and tart as a Granny Smith apple, kombucha is a naturally fermented beverage infused with probiotics and enzymes that delivers a cidery flavor and a kick of fizziness. The result is a slightly sweet and slightly sour beverage containing a long list of amino acids, B vitamins, and live probiotics and enzymes.

You don't want to guzzle down a bottle of kombucha—which has also become widely available in natural food stores in the last decade—on a hot summer's day. Instead, you sip slowly. I've become a kombucha fan who'll drink as many as two or three bottles per day, if I'm in the mood.

There's another fermented beverage that I want to mention but is one that's not as easy to find. I'm referring to kvass (pronounced *kuh-VAHSS*), which is reputed to be Russian in origin. A fermented beverage made from rye, barley, or beets, kvass tastes a bit like beer or ale—but this cultured beverage isn't alcoholic. Those who appreciate kvass say that opening a bottle of kvass releases a fragrant bouquet reminiscent of freshly baked bread cooling on a windowsill. Kvass made from veggies is now available in health food stores but is certainly an acquired taste.

If there's one fermented beverage that's too sour to drink straight out of the bottle, that would be apple cider vinegar, the tartest of all fermented beverages. (I've taken a few apple cider vinegar shots in the past, so I speak from experience.) When used to make salad dressing, added to marinades, or mixed in purified water, apple cider vinegar helps the body balance its pH levels, which is critical for the health of your internal environment.

Apple cider vinegar was born out of necessity when farmers had too many apples on trees to bring to market during the harvest season. They had to do something with their bushels of apples besides making apple juice, apple cider, and applesauce!

Orchard farmers discovered that adding sugar and yeast to the squeezed liquid of crushed apples initiated a fermentation process that turned the sugar into alcohol. During a second round of fermentation, the alcohol was converted by acetic acid-forming bacteria into vinegar. The word *vinegar* comes from the French, meaning "sour wine."

Apple cider vinegar gets its "pucker power" from acetic acid. Apple cider vinegar contains a plethora of minerals—potassium, phosphorus, calcium, magnesium, and natural silicon as well as pectin and tartaric acid. One of apple cider vinegar's greatest health attributes is how it helps the body maintain its pH balance, starting with the colon, which should be slightly acidic for optimal health.

Apple cider vinegar has been traditionally used for every health system and organ of the body. There's even clinical research with studies showing apple cider vinegar supporting blood sugar levels and a healthy immune system, along with germ-fighting properties and improving digestion and assimilation.

I first heard about the incredible health benefits of apple cider vinegar through a Vermont physician named D.C. Jarvis, M.D., who injected the lore of folk medicine into his practice. His book, *Folk Medicine*, has sold over three million copies during the last fifty years, and even today you still see *Folk Medicine* featured on end cap displays in health food stores. Apple cider vinegar is one of the most beloved substances in natural health history.

For years, I've made my own salad dressing that mixes apple cider vinegar with extra-virgin olive oil, high-mineral sea salt, herbs, and spices. I consume a lot of salad, so I appreciate the healing cleansing properties of my homemade salad dressing.

INTRODUCING HERBAL FERMENTATION

My long history with apple cider vinegar brought a compelling thought to mind recently, and it went like this: Could I apply the magic of apple cider vinegar to other plant-based substances such as herbs, taking the fermentation concept beyond apples and applying it to botanicals—plants valued for their medicinal or therapeutic properties?

I knew that herbs have been around for as long as fermentation. Whether dating back to ancient Egypt, the practice of Ayurveda in India, traditional Chinese herbs, as well as the hundreds of references to herbs and spices in the Bible, herbs have a long tradition in cultures around the world. The use of herbs—whether it's from a root such as ginger, a leaf such as holy basil, or a piece of bark such as cinnamon—to promote wellness is backed up by plenty of hard science.

As I studied herbal extracts, however, I learned that the typical manufacturing process applies heat and employs harsh chemical solvents, including alcohol—agents that fundamentally change their properties. Hexane, one of the most commonly used solvents, kills enzymes and beneficial microorganisms. Alcohol adulterates the herbal properties, and adding heat zaps beneficial enzymes and microorganisms as well.

The entire chemical extraction process was an anomaly to me. I didn't see the wisdom in bench scientists focusing on extracting the "healthy" compounds in herbs or herbal plants when there had to be other nutrients left behind that could offer their own health benefits. My premise was that the "whole plant" provides the health benefit, not just one, two, or three isolated compounds present in the substance.

My desire to deliver the immense benefits of herbs and spices in a form the body can truly utilize became a challenge.

But alas, that challenge was about to be overcome.

11

BIBLICAL BOTANICALS

I love how I can read Scripture and learn something new each and every time.

If you pay close attention, you'll read about plenty of herbs and spices in the Bible, which adds to the richness of God's Word just as those herbs and spices added zest and health benefits to those who lived at that time.

Herbs and spices were grown in Palestine as well as neighboring Syria and Egypt and formed a basis of trade in ancient times. One of the first mentions of herbs and spices happens in the Old Testament in Exodus 12:8 when the Hebrews were instructed to kill an unblemished lamb, take some of the blood and put it on their doorposts, and then consume roasted lamb with unleavened bread and "bitter herbs."

Good thing the Hebrews weren't hooked on sweet or salty foods like we are.

Moses was told to make a holy anointing oil out of myrrh, cinnamon, sweet-smelling cane, cassia, and olive oil. Myrrh is referred to again in Matthew 2 when the Three Kings visited the infant Jesus and presented gifts to him—gold, frankincense, and myrrh. And, more soberly, myrrh is mentioned again in John 19 when Joseph of Arimathea asked for the body of Jesus following His death by crucifixion and arrived with Nicodemus, "bringing a mixture of myrrh and aloes, about a hundred pounds" (John 19:39).

Herbs and spices have been prized as powerful health agents by cultures around the world for centuries. Herbs can be taken as teas, juices, baths, extracts, oils, and tinctures and are being relied upon by a growing number of Americans for the health of their families. Likewise, spices have aromatic properties that are used to season or flavor foods as well as convey health benefits.

Technically, herbs come from a plant or a part of a plant while most spices are derived from bark, such as cinnamon or nutmeg, or a root in the case of turmeric. But can herbs be spices and spices be herbs? The answer is *yes* because many herbs can flavor foods while a lot of spices can be used for health purposes, but herbs and spices are both superstars in their own right.

Let me share some of my favorite herbs and spices, which include tea, the most widely consumed beverage in the world after water. The Chinese have a saying about tea: "Better to be deprived of food for three days, than of tea for one."

All true varieties of tea come from the leaves of a single evergreen plant, *Camellia sinensis*. (Herbal teas such as chamomile and peppermint should really be called herbal infusions as they don't contain any true tea.) During harvest time, tea leaves are picked, rolled, dried, and heated. The type of tea depends on how the leaves are processed. Green and white teas are non-fermented and are the freshest. Black teas are the most fermented, which is worth noting. Oolong teas are in between.

Teas often come in teabags, which most Americans prefer, but teas also come in loose leaf forms, which mean the loose teas must be steeped in hot water for three to a five minutes, then filtered out to create an *infusion* or *decoction*.

Green tea accounts for 20 percent of the global tea market, while black tea (or green tea that has been subjected to additional processing that ferments the leaves) accounts for about 78 percent. When consuming hot tea, organic honey or evaporated coconut nectar should be used as a sweetener, and tea is best served warm.

And just what makes tea so special? The secret behind tea lies in its high content of a class of health-promoting agents collectively known as polyphenols or flavonoids—specifically the group known as catechins.

Since I'm on the subject, tea should come from organic sources. While hot tea infusions can be wonderful, my favorite use of black tea is in the fermented beverage known as kombucha that unlocks the best of tea's powerful benefits.

Herbal infusions made from daisy-like chamomile flowers have been often consumed as an after-dinner beverage to settle stomachs and help with digestion. Others believe chamomile has mild sedative properties, which help them fall asleep.

There are literally thousands of herbs and spices being used somewhere in the world. I'm only going to list a handful, but here are a few that I wanted to call to your attention to, in alphabetical order:

↙ **Cinnamon** is a fragrant spice that's been used since biblical times for its health and culinary properties. The Romans used cinnamon to take the edge off their strong, bitter wine, and the Greeks used it to season their meat and vegetables. The exotic, sweet-flavored spice comes from the outer brown bark of Cinnamomum trees.

Americans love cinnamon; all you have to do is walk around a mall on a Saturday afternoon and breathe in the crisp smell of cinnamon wafting from the ovens at cinnamon bun shops and pretzel outlets.

↙ **Cumin** is another delightful spice with a nutty, pepper flavor produced from small, potent seeds that are longitudinally ridged and yellow/brown in color. Cumin was so popular in the Middle Ages that soldiers in Europe marched off to war with loaves of cumin bread in their satchels. The spice originated in Egypt and has a long history as supporting digestive issues by stimulating the liver to secrete more bile, which aids in the breakdown of fats and the absorption of nutrients. Cumin is also an excellent source of iron, which is instrumental in the health of red blood cells.

↙ **Dandelion** may be viewed as a pesky weed in your backyard lawn, but this valuable herb can be used as a food or a health-supporting agent. When dandelion leaves decorate any salad, this herb contributes to urinary tract and digestive health.

↙ **Echinacea**, a perennial plant that is slightly spiky and has large purple to pink flowers, comes from the dry prairies and open woodlands of the Great Plains region. It was the most widely used medicinal plant for Native Americans before the arrival of European explorers and settlers. This herb is ultra popular to support seasonal wellness.

↙ **Ginger,** the world's most widely cultivated spice, appears in countless varieties, shapes, and sizes. This pungent spice comes from the underground stem of the *Zingiber offinale* plant that is often found in India, China, Mexico, and several other countries.

Each variety of ginger possesses its own distinctive flavor and aroma, and all you have to do is lean down toward a cutting board and take in a sharp whiff of its sweet perfumed sharpness to encounter one of the most unique sensory experiences you'll ever come across. The special flavor of ginger adds bite to Asian dishes as well as to vegetable sides.

Ginger has a historical tradition of promoting gastrointestinal health and supporting numerous systems of the body, including fighting occasional nausea. In addition, ginger contains potent compounds called *gingerols*, which support healthy inflammation response and promote healthy joints, ligaments, and tendons.

↙ **Holy basil** is a culinary herb grown in profusion around Hindu temples, which explains why it's revered in India and used in Ayurveda. The Hindu name for holy basil, *Tulasi* or *Tulsi*, means "the incomparable one."

In the kitchen, holy basil is added to stir-fry dishes and spicy soups because of its sharp, peppery taste. Chefs call this herb "hot basil" and appreciate how its flavor intensifies as heat is applied. Indian families regard holy basil as a purifying agent for both the mind and the body, which explains why this herb is held in high regard in India.

↙ **Hyssop** is one of the better-known plants of the Bible, referred to twelve times in Scripture. "Purge me with hyssop, and I shall be clean; wash me, and I shall be whiter than snow" (Psalm 51:7).

Hyssop is a common herb that grows to about two feet tall and about a foot wide with beautiful purple-blue flowers and a strong minty smell. Its name in Hebrew is *azob*, which literally means "holy herb."

I've always liked using hyssop in its essential oil form. I love taking hot, dry saunas and steam showers, and while I'm sitting inside, I'll rub a few drops of essential oil of hyssop into my palms, then cup my hands over my mouth and nose and inhale. I also love to rub drops of the oil on my feet, which circulates the compounds throughout the body.

A drop or two of an essential oil such as hyssop, cinnamon, lavender, or frankincense stimulates the olfactory nerves and improves the physical and emotional health of our bodies.

𝕃 **Milk thistle** gets its name from the milky white sap that comes from the leaves of this stout plant native to the Mediterranean region. Milk thistle is one of the most popular herbs for the support of liver health and detoxification.

𝕃 **Oregano** is a beautiful herb native to the Mediterranean and has been an important ingredient for cooking in Greece, Italy, and Egypt for centuries. Oregano is one of the few herbs that actually increases in pungency and flavor once it's dried. Oregano supports healthy microbial balance throughout the body.

𝕃 **Turmeric,** which comes from a perennial plant, is a cousin of ginger and a pungent Indian spice that imparts a vivid yellow color. Turmeric has gained significant popularity as a powerful source of antioxidants and is the ingredient in mustard that gives the condiment its famous yellow color.

𝕃 **Thyme** is a delicate herb with a penetrating fragrance that's a wonderful addition to any kitchen spice rack and used to season stock, stews, and soups. Thyme contains certain flavonoids with powerful antioxidant capacity and is a good source of calcium and dietary fiber when consumed whole.

HERBAL EXTRACTIONS

I've never needed any convincing that herbs and spices have amazing properties, although it seems herbal folk remedies were much more effective in the past.

Why is that? Could it be that our ability to digest, assimilate, and fully utilize these nutrients and compounds has been compromised due to the toxins in our food supply and environment?

We don't have a good answer yet, but that doesn't mean we shouldn't stop seeking the health benefits that herbs and spices can offer us. How to successfully access those health benefits is a challenge, though.

I thought there must be a way to develop an effective delivery system to help herbs express their full potential within the body. After more than a decade of trying, I believe I've found the solution—a live food fermentation process called "bio-transformation."

I've long been a champion of fermentation—the natural preservation and pre-digestion of foods utilizing beneficial bacteria, yeast, and even mold. If fermentation could preserve and improve the vitality of food, then in my mind, fermentation of botanicals would certainly have merit.

When it came to unlocking the full spectrum of benefits found in herbs and spices, bio-transformation turned out to be a perfect process. We found that a long cycle of fermentation not only unlocked the full spectrum of active compounds in herbs, but also a bevy of other nutrients were either enhanced or created. As we began to consume the fruits or rather the herbs of our labor, I could feel the benefits of these amazing botanicals in a way I never had before.

I decided to call these fermented herbal extracts "Terrain Living Herbals," and they are a synergistic combination of organic botanicals infused with ancient symbiotic microorganisms.

Just as it takes a considerable length of time for grapes to ferment into a fine wine, we found that the fermentation process was something you couldn't rush either. All Terrain Living Herbals undergo a fermentation process that lasts three to eight months and utilizes ancient symbiotic cultures to produce enzymes, organic acids, and bioactive compounds to support digestive and immune system health.

At the time of this writing, there are sixteen different Terrain Living Herbal formulas containing vitamins, probiotics, enzymes, and antioxidants that will help you rebuild your inner ecosystem and replenish key nutrients that your body craves. I believe the secret to building a strong terrain can be found in adapting sweet- and salt-loving taste buds to these sour-tasting liquid herbal tonics made from organic botanicals.

Yes, Terrain Living Herbals impart a sour taste, but when it comes to boosting your body's terrain, *sour* is the secret.

Does this mean you have to pucker up every time you consume them? Not at all. You can mitigate the sour taste of living herbal botanicals such as turmeric and milk thistle by diluting them in water, juice, tea, or veggie juice. I just consumed 30 milliliters or two tablespoons of Terrain Sacred Herbs in vegetable juice as I was writing this chapter, and it was awesome. You can try Terrain Turmeric in a curry sauce or Terrain Kombucha Black Tea in any beverage.

Terrain Living Herbals are best consumed upon waking, before sleep, and prior to the largest meal of the day to support digestive function, so now let me introduce you to Terrain Living Herbals by Beyond Organic:

↙ **Terrain Sacred Herbs** is a combination of turmeric and holy basil, two plants native to India and South Asia. When I was in India in 2012, I saw firsthand how turmeric and holy basil were considered "sacred" and have been treasured for thousands of years within Ayurvedic herbalism in India. The traditional health system of India for thousands of years, Ayurveda emphasizes re-establishing balance in the body through diet, lifestyle, exercise, and body cleansing. Turmeric and holy basil are superstar botanicals, which makes Terrain Sacred Herbs a great foundational herbal formula for everyone.

Terrain Sacred Herbs, which supports blood sugar levels in the normal range as well as the maintenance of healthy cholesterol levels, is probably my favorite Terrain Herbal formula.

↙ **Terrain Turmeric** provides the foundational benefits of healthy metabolism, digestion, and balanced pH levels in the body while supporting healthy joint function and healthy skin by providing antioxidants to help support your cells against oxidative stress due to free radicals. Terrain Turmeric also supports cardiovascular health.

↙ **Terrain Holy Basil** supports a positive stress response and cellular health while promoting a calm and balanced mood and healthy energy levels.

↙ **Terrain Ginger** supports cardiovascular function and a healthy inflammation response while also supporting healthy intestinal function including alleviating occasional nausea.

↙ **Terrain Oregano** supports respiratory health and healthy immune system function while maintaining a healthy inflammatory response to seasonal stressors.

⚘ **Terrain Peppermint** supports healthy digestion and brain function and has a very distinct minty taste.

⚘ **Terrain Milk Thistle** supports healthy liver function and detoxification as well as healthy kidney and gallbladder function while promoting healthy skin.

⚘ **Terrain Echinacea** supports a healthy immune system response, maintains a healthy inflammatory response to seasonal stressors, and promotes the healthy drainage of the lymphatic system.

⚘ **Terrain Kombucha Black Tea** is a slightly sour beverage with an effervescent taste. Terrain Kombucha Black Tea supports healthy energy levels and the body's natural detoxification efforts while providing antioxidants that can help support your cells against excessive oxidation and free radicals.

⚘ **Terrain Cinnamon** supports healthy blood sugar levels, healthy microbial balance, and imparts a nice flavor and a warming sensation.

⚘ **Terrain Star Anise** helps support immune system function and digestive health. Star Anise is the fruit of a small evergreen tree native to southwest China, so these star-shaped fruits with a licorice taste are not well known in this country. Star anise pairs well with fruit and is used to flavor teas, marinades, and soups.

⚘ **Terrain Garlic** supports healthy microorganism balance within the body. Garlic, commonly used in American kitchens, has an intense and unique flavor that's a welcome addition to sauces, marinades, soups, and cooked meats. Garlic has shown an ability to support healthy immune system function as well as cardiovascular health, particularly in the area of blood pressure.

⚘ **Terrain American Ginseng** supports healthy energy levels and enables the body to better adapt to stressors. Ginseng, a root, has been prized by ancient emperors as an energy and vitality tonic.

⚘ **Terrain Maca** brings you a health secret from the high-altitude Andes mountains in South America. Maca, a tuber, has been used to support healthy hormone function in both men and women.

⚘ **Terrain Ashwagandha** rounds out arguably the top three most popular herbs in the subcontinent of India (along with turmeric and holy basil).

Ashwagandha is considered an adaptogenic herb that supports multiple functions and systems of the body to resist the many stressors of life.

↙ **Terrain Coffee** promotes healthy energy levels within the body. Believe it or not, coffee is the number-one source of antioxidants in this country, but that's because so much coffee is poured each day. Coffee's notable antioxidants are chlorogenic acid and caffeic acid, which help support healthy blood sugar levels and cardiovascular health.

There's not a single person on this planet who couldn't benefit from this cornucopia of herbal botanicals gathered from around the world. You'll experience the fullness of herbal nutrition without alcohol extractions, high heat, or chemicals. You're going to consume herbal nutrition as it was designed through a delivery system that starts with the bio-transformation fermentation process.

ADVANCED PROTOCOLS

If you're looking to experience the unique combination of the sour secret and biblical botanicals, here are a dozen ways and combinations to use Terrain Living Herbals:

For healthy digestion, I encourage you to consume 30 milliliters of Terrain Sacred Herbs first thing in the morning in 16 ounces of purified water. This will wake up your digestive tract.

Before dinner, I recommend 30 milliliters of Terrain Peppermint mixed in 16 ounces of water ten to twenty minutes before a meal. This will stimulate your gastric juices and get you ready to utilize the nutrition that is in that meal.

Before bed, I encourage you to consume 30 milliliters of Terrain Ginger in water to support healthy digestion and a healthy inflammation response, which will allow your sleep to be transformative.

For daily immune system support, start with 30 milliliters of Terrain Sacred Herbs in 16 ounces of purified water when you wake up. At dinner time, mix 30 milliliters of Terrain Garlic in water to support healthy immune system function. Before bedtime, consume 30 milliliters of Terrain Kombucha Black Tea in water to support the body's detoxification efforts.

For seasonal immune support, I encourage you to consume 30 milliliters of Terrain Star Anise first thing in the morning in 16 ounces of purified water. Before dinner, I recommend 30 milliliters of Terrain Oregano mixed in 16 ounces of water ten to twenty minutes before a meal. Before bed, I encourage you to consume 30 milliliters of Terrain Echinacea for unparalleled immune system support.

For healthy inflammation, including supporting joints, ligaments, and tendons, and improving flexibility, start with 30 milliliters of Terrain Turmeric first thing in the morning in 16 ounces of purified water.

Before dinner, I recommend 30 milliliters of Terrain Ginger mixed in 16 ounces of water ten to twenty minutes before a meal. This will stimulate your gastric juices and get you ready to utilize the nutrition that is in that meal.

Before bed, probably an hour before, I encourage you to consume 30 milliliters of Terrain Holy Basil in water to support healthy digestion and healthy inflammation response and to boost your mood, which will allow your sleep to be transformative.

This is a powerful protocol.

For energy, start with 30 milliliters of Terrain Coffee in 16 ounces of purified water upon waking up. Before dinner, consume 30 milliliters of Terrain Kombucha Black Tea in water, and thirty to sixty minutes before bed, take 30 milliliters of Terrain American Ginseng to provide a boost to the organs and systems of your body.

For brain health, I suggest beginning the day with 30 milliliters of Terrain Ginseng in 16 ounces of purified water after rising. Before dinner, take 30 milliliters of Terrain Peppermint followed by 30 milliliters of Terrain Holy Basil before bedtime.

For healthy metabolism, start with Terrain Coffee by mixing thirty milliliters in water. Before dinner, take 30 milliliters of Terrain Kombucha Black Tea followed by 30 milliliters of Terrain Ashwagandha before you fall asleep.

To support healthy detoxification, begin the day with 30 milliliters of Terrain Garlic in 16 ounces of purified water when you wake up. At dinner time, mix 30 milliliters of Terrain Milk Thistle in water to support detoxification as well as healthy kidney and gallbladder function. Before bedtime, consume 30 milliliters of Terrain Kombucha Black Tea in water to also support the body's natural detoxification efforts.

For healthy skin, I recommend you to consume 30 milliliters of Terrain Turmeric first thing in the morning in 16 ounces of purified water to provide antioxidants that will help support your cells. Before dinner, I recommend 30 milliliters of Terrain Cinnamon mixed in water ten to twenty minutes before a meal. Before bedtime, consume 30 milliliters of Terrain Holy Basil in water to also support cellular health as well as healthy skin.

For blood sugar support, get the day going with 30 milliliters of Terrain Coffee in 16 ounces of purified water when you wake up. At dinner time, mix 30 milliliters of Terrain Cinnamon in water to support detoxification as well as healthy kidney and gallbladder function. Before bedtime, consume 30 milliliters of Terrain Sacred Herbs in water to help you maintain blood sugar levels.

To support healthy cardiovascular function, I encourage you to consume 30 milliliters of Terrain Garlic first thing in the morning in 16 ounces of purified water. Before dinner, I recommend 30 milliliters of Terrain Cinnamon mixed in water ten to twenty minutes before a meal. Before bed, probably an hour before, I encourage you to consume 30 milliliters of Terrain Sacred Herbs in water to support the cardiovascular system.

To support healthy cholesterol levels, begin with Terrain Sacred Herbs after waking up, mixing 30 milliliters in 16 ounces of purified water. Before dinner, consume 30 milliliters of Terrain Garlic in water. An hour before bed, finish the day with 30 milliliters of Terrain Kombucha Black Tea, which provides antioxidants to help support your cells against excessive oxidation and free radicals.

I want you to remember one thing about Terrain Living Herbals. As you unlock the secret of sour, your body will change, as well as your taste buds. You will grow to enjoy these zero calorie, zero sugar, high probiotic, antioxidant- and enzyme-rich herbal infusions.

Once that happens, you've truly transformed your terrain.

12

THE BODY ELECTRIC

As much as modern medicine and science can tell us about the inner workings of the body, we've only scratched the surface of understanding the mind-blowing complexity of the cells, tissues, organs, joints, cartilage, muscles, the digestive tract, the cardiovascular system, and the brain—all of which reflect the unfathomable intelligence of the skillful designer, God Himself.

You start with the scientific fact that every human being is composed of roughly 100 trillion cells. Try getting your head around that number.

Next, consider what each of these minute cells—they're way smaller than the width of a human hair—have to do on a 24/7 basis. At any given time, each cell has an important task to do, from creating and using energy to manufacturing proteins to responding to environmental cues. Other cells build skin and bone, some pump out hormones, and others produce antibodies. The number of tasks is endless.

The nervous system regulates all the body's activities and stimulates the parts of the body—from the simplest cells to the complex digestive system to the muscles and joints—by nerve impulses, which can travel up to speeds of 100 meters per second.

Nerve impulses—neurons—travel in and between the cells much like electric currents travel through telephone wires. Minerals such as sodium, potassium, magnesium, and calcium are electrolytes that dissolve in water and help carry an electrical charge. The body needs these electrolytes to transport nutrients and waste matter and to maintain electrical impulses.

For example, let's say you have an itch on your scalp. Your brain feels the itch and transmits a message to the muscles in your right arm and hand to go find that itch and give it a scratch. Neurons use electrically charged particles known as ions to communicate between the brain and your right arm.

Two of the most important ions in your nervous system are sodium and potassium. The following description is vastly simplifying things, but encasing each cell of the body is a special "pump" that allows sodium or potassium ions to move in and out of the cells. Each time one of these electrolytes makes a move, an electrical charge is produced. The sodium-potassium pump also responds to a "request line" from the nervous system to help maintain vital systems in the body and plays a crucial role in the brain, nervous system, and muscles, all of which require electrical signals for communication.

Sodium is the major positive ion in the fluid *outside* the cells while potassium is the major positive ion *inside* the cells. Proper electrolyte balance in the cells is very important for proper cellular function and good health. Sodium is essential for hydration since it pumps water and nutrients into the cells, and potassium pumps waste products out of the cells.

So what happens when that balance is out of whack? Because of our sodium-rich diets, we're more likely to have too much sodium outside the cells, waiting to pass through the pump and to mix with the positive potassium ions inside the cells. The extra sodium means we're holding excess stagnant fluid in the body, which is a primary cause of elevated blood pressure. When either sodium or potassium levels become imbalanced, the kidneys may expend the other electrolyte to maintain an equilibrium.

Maintaining the right sodium to potassium balance is rarely talked about in health circles, but it should be. Even though everyone has heard that high cholesterol levels have a correlation to cardiovascular health, I doubt one in 10,000 people are aware that the ratio of sodium to potassium in and outside the cell is one of the most important numbers that exists for overall health and detoxification.

Most Americans consume ten times as much sodium as they do potassium each day, for a ratio of 10:1, but that ratio needs to be drastically altered.

We should receive twice as much potassium as we do sodium. That means a normal, healthy ratio of sodium to potassium within the extracellular and intracellular fluid should be around 1:2. This would be best accomplished by consuming *fewer* high-sodium foods and *more* potassium-rich foods in our diets.

You can't blame our high salt intake on the naturally occurring sodium in healthy foods, which is just 5 percent of our sodium intake. But you can sure point a finger at the sodium intake coming from the added salt found in processed foods (45 percent) and adding salt during cooking of foods (another 45 percent). The remaining 5 percent comes from condiments such as ketchup and mustard.

When you eat the standard American diet, with its reliance on salty chips, double-decker hamburgers, and garlic fries, this tilts the playing field toward an excess of sodium inside the body. When the ratio of potassium ions in the cells is overwhelmed by the sodium ions, there's an inability to properly remove toxins from the body, which can lead to health challenges.

I've heard about this sodium/potassium ratio for years because of Dr. Paul Eck, an early pioneer in metabolic nutrition who relied on information gained from a mineral analysis of hair samples taken from his patients.

Back in the 1970s, Dr. Eck developed a laboratory test for human hair that measured twenty or so minerals, including sodium, potassium, magnesium, calcium, zinc, and iron. From a half dozen small cuttings of hair from the back of the head, Dr. Eck believed he could evaluate adrenal function, thyroid function, and the body's ability to detoxify heavy metals from the results.

For instance, Dr. Eck theorized:

- An imbalanced ratio of sodium to potassium suggests problems with the adrenal glands, blood pressure, and immune system.

- An imbalanced radio of calcium to magnesium suggests problems with blood sugar.

- An imbalanced ratio of calcium to potassium suggests thyroid problems.

When your sodium/potassium ratio is imbalanced, then you are simply unable to cleanse the body of toxins effectively. Without effective cleansing, you can't truly rebuild your body.

What About Taking Potassium Supplements?

So, if the need for dietary potassium is so clear, why don't I recommend potassium supplements?

Answer: Because the U.S. Food and Drug Administration tightly regulates potassium supplements, and the allowable dose provides only a limited amount of the mineral per serving. In fact, many forms of potassium are available only at pharmacies with a prescription. Injectable or infused potassium can only be administered by or under the supervision of a doctor. Perhaps the FDA is being careful because there is evidence that potassium can be lethal even in small doses, causing your heart to stop cold. (Heart surgeons use a special potassium solution to paralyze the heart at the start of their surgical procedures.)

Over-the-counter potassium supplements are limited by the FDA to a dose of 99 milligrams, yet the recommended daily allowance is 4,700 milligrams, so one capsule is only around 2 percent of the RDA. Thus, taking one potassium supplement per day—the recommended amount—would barely add to your potassium intake. Those who do take a 99-milligram dose of potassium often complain of having a metallic taste in the mouth.

That's further proof that the best way to bring up your potassium level is to consume foods and beverages rich in this important electrolyte.

Yes, consuming less sodium will improve your sodium/potassium ratio, but the best way to improve your ratio is to *increase* the amount of potassium in your diet. You can take a big step toward improving your sodium/potassium ratio when you embark on the 10-Day Daniel Diet, which will flood your body with potassium and thereby remove excess sodium. Since there is no added salt included during the ten-day diet, your body can "reset" your ratio.

When the Daniel Diet is over and you return to eating regular meals—hopefully within a tighter time window of six to eight hours—it's important to consume potassium-rich cleansing beverages during the cleansing period and potassium-rich fruits and vegetables during the building or eating time. You should also replace the regular table salt in your pantry with high mineral sea salt.

The key to a properly wired "body electric" may rest on how well you're able to make these dietary changes.

THINK POTASSIUM

Because potassium populates the inside of the cell membrane, it's the most important electrolyte in the human cells. This mineral is essential for the functioning of the heart and kidneys and the conversion of blood sugar into glycogen, which is the storage form of blood sugar found in the liver and the muscles.

A potassium shortage means a lower level of stored glycogen. The body calls upon its stores of glycogen during times of exercise, so when there's a potassium deficiency, you'll experience fatigue, muscle weakness, and cramps. That's why potassium-rich bananas are especially popular on the tennis court, where Rafael Nadal and Maria Sharapova devour them during changeovers. Tour de France cyclists often find a banana when handed their lunch bags as they pedal through the French countryside. Potassium is the electrolyte mineral that seeps out of their pores when they work up a good sweat.

Even if you're just a weekend warrior—or someone whose idea of exercise is taking the stairs to work—you still need plenty of potassium. A potassium deficit will leave you feeling fatigued and out of it. Arm and leg cramps are common. Lesser known symptoms include constipation, excessive thirst, excessive urination, and nausea.

Consuming a variety of foods and beverages rich in potassium is the best way to make sure your cells have enough to keep everything running well and on schedule. Potassium's recommended daily allowance of 4,700 milligrams is a number that everyone should aim for. The average American doesn't even receive a fourth of that amount.

Here's a list of the potassium content in various foods, in milligrams, per serving. (And look at how much potassium just half an avocado has!)

Fresh vegetables:

- potato (medium-sized): 782 milligrams

- avocado (half): 680 milligrams

- lima beans (cooked, half cup): 581 milligrams

- raw tomato (medium-sized): 444 milligrams

- spinach (cooked, half cup): 292 milligrams

- asparagus (cooked, half cup): 165 milligrams

- corn (half cup): 136 milligrams

Fresh fruits:

- banana (medium): 440 milligrams

- cantaloupe (half): 341 milligrams

- dried apricots (dried, half cup): 318 milligrams

- peach (medium): 308 milligrams

- orange (medium): 263 milligrams

- apple (medium): 182 milligrams

- plums (five): 150 milligrams

- strawberries (half cup): 122 milligrams

Unprocessed meats (per three ounces):

- chicken: 350 milligrams

- lamb: 241 milligrams

- beef: 224 milligrams

Fish (per three ounces):

- flounder: 498 milligrams

- salmon: 378 milligrams

- cod: 345 milligrams

- haddock: 297 milligrams

- tuna: 225 milligrams

There's another food—actually, it's a beverage—that's rich in potassium, low in sodium, and free of fat and cholesterol—coconut water. In the last five years, coconut water has become extremely popular even in regular supermarkets, where the packaging evokes the healthiness of the South Pacific by showing palm trees waving in sunny tropical breezes. During a recent trip to New York City, I was surprised to see young green coconuts, with tops sheared off and a straw poking out, being hawked on the streets of Manhattan.

There's no doubt that coconut water packs a potassium punch and helps balance sodium and potassium levels. Unfortunately, the potassium in coconut water is provided to the exclusion of sodium, which can push the balance out of whack the other way, leading to excess detoxification.

I am a fan of consuming coconut water provided that it is consumed fresh from the coconut. Consuming coconut water from a carton is less desirable since the product has been processed with excessive heat, destroying the enzymes.

There is a beverage, though, that tops coconut water when it comes to balancing the sodium and potassium ratio. I'm talking about whey or cultured whey, which I introduced in Chapter 2, "After the Cleanse."

When it comes to improving the ratio of sodium to potassium in the body, cultured whey is really the way to go.

A GOLDEN LIQUID

You've got to love the innocence of an English nursery rhyme that's been around for more than two hundred years:

Little Miss Muffet sat on a tuffet, eating her curds and whey....

During the cheese-production process, whey is the resulting liquid after curds are separated from milk to make cheese. I still remember the first time I saw an almost glowing golden liquid separating from the cheese at the Beyond Organic dairy processing center in southern Missouri.

Most people have heard of whey because they include a scoop of whey protein in their smoothies, even though they really don't know much about its origins. Whey protein isn't a necessarily a food but rather an isolated fraction of whey that is fine to use as a protein supplement as long as it comes from pasture-fed cattle that are naturally raised. Unfortunately, most whey protein comes from conventionally raised cattle that are exposed to hormones and antibiotics and fed GMO grains.

What makes golden whey so beneficial is the unique balance of organically bound electrolytes it contains. In fact, whey provides what I believe to be the best source of naturally occurring sodium and potassium—both in the correct ratio for cellular health. There's also another wonderful electrolyte in whey—acidified and organically bound calcium. Live probiotics, B vitamins, and other key nutrients are contained in whey as well. Talk about an amazing resource to help your cells function properly.

Historically, whey has been prized for its ability to support the body's health in four unique ways:

- Whey, with its natural blend of sodium and potassium, stimulates intestinal peristalsis to support healthy bowel function.

- Whey, with its probiotics, organic acids, and sugars that feed probiotics, supports intestinal flora.

- Whey hydrates the cells of the body.

- Whey contains a high percentage of water and organically bound minerals to support elimination via the liver, kidneys, and colon.

These four factors attest to whey being an incredible agent to support cleansing and detoxification on a daily basis. I first learned about whey from one of my health mentors, Bud Keith, who introduced me to the concept of biblical eating. Cultured whey was an important part of the health plan he introduced me to when I traveled to San Diego in search of my own health transformation.

Another mentor of mine, Dr. Bernard Jensen, further explained the benefits of whey. I'll never forget the last time I saw him. It was the late 1990s, and Dr. Jensen was nearing the end of his life at the famed Hidden Valley Health Ranch he founded on one hundred acres of lush, rolling foothills near the Southern California city of Escondido.

During the 1950s and 1960s, Hidden Valley Health Ranch gained a reputation as a special healing place. Patients came from around the world seeking help. Heads of state, sports figures, Hollywood celebrities, and ordinary folks suffering from arthritis, cancer, weight disorders, and other chronic and degenerative diseases stayed at Hidden Valley seeking to transform their health.

Dr. Jensen saw more than 350,000 patients in his life and was a prolific author of more than fifty books, preaching mainly on the topic of cleansing and detoxification. The practice of cleansing the digestive system, lungs, kidneys, and liver should be a routine part of everyone's health care strategy, he said.

When I visited him that afternoon, he was ninety-two years old. He smiled and sat up in his bed. "Get a pad and a pen," he said, summoning strength. "Here are the most important things you need to know about health."

I distinctly remember Dr. Jensen talking about whey as being beneficial for every system in the body. He recommended whey as an ideal tool to prevent or correct diet-caused mineral deficiencies. Cleansing, he emphasized, is important because one of the body's natural ways of staying healthy is its ability to detoxify itself.

I took notes, but more importantly, his words stayed with me. I knew he was right about detoxification. Every day, we are exposed to some type of toxin, whether it be environmental pollution, chemicals found in our drinking water or food, secondhand cigarette smoke, or household cleaning products. Excessive toxicity has been linked to many conditions such as digestive issues, hormonal imbalances, fatigue, joint discomfort, and even brain fog. Toxins accumulate in our cells—despite the cells' best attempts to keep them from penetrating the cell membrane—which makes it all the more imperative to cleanse our bodies and our cells on a regular basis.

True cleansing starts at the cellular level. A healthy cell is able to bring nutrients in and push toxins out, a process made easier because cells are 60 percent water. If you imagine your cells as a bunch of little lakes, with springs feeding into the lakes and flushing out existing water downstream, a healthy cell is able to receive nutrients (such as fresh spring water) and expel waste (like flushing stagnant water downstream).

Because cells contain so much fluid, cleansing *beverages* are even more effective than cleansing foods in my opinion. As mentioned previously, I first experienced the benefits of cultured whey in San Diego while being introduced to the health plan I would later call *The Maker's Diet*. I often consumed as many as two or three 16-ounce bottles of this tart yet tasty beverage daily to boost my probiotic intake.

I was reintroduced to cultured whey on my first trip to Switzerland ten years ago. My wife, Nicki, and I—this was before kids—were visiting the Swiss alpine village of Kandersteg, known for its hiking trails and awesome views of snow-topped peaks, even in summer.

Nicki and I were strolling past shops in the center of the village when I noticed a product called Molkosan in a window display. Intrigued, I made inquiries and learned that Molkosan was a cultured whey concentrate developed by the famed Swiss naturopathic doctor Alfred Vogel. I was told the "cheese water" had an abundance of powerful but rare nutrients and compounds to support good health, influencing the digestive tract and hence the immune system in positive ways.

Of course, I had to try a bottle. Yes, the taste was definitely sour, but I appreciated the tangy freshness and the health benefits of Molkosan, which was manufactured in the Appenzell farming region of Switzerland. I also made a mental note to investigate the health properties of cultured whey further.

Fast forward to the present day and our Beyond Organic dairy center in southern Missouri. During the process of making our raw, GreenFed cheese, we produce organic whey and then culture or ferment it with powerful probiotics. This cultured whey has become the foundation of our beverage known as SueroViv. The name is a combination of *suero* (which is Spanish for whey) and *viv* (which is a French way of saying "life"). So SueroViv means "whey of life."

I introduced this certified organic, alkalizing cultured whey beverage in Chapter 2, calling it a "secret weapon" when undergoing your monthly three-day cleanse. While I recommend consuming cultured whey daily during the cleansing period, SueroViv shines as the sole nourishment during the weekly one-day cleanse (on Cleanse Day Wednesday) and the monthly three-day cleanse. I call this partial fast the "Suero Cleanse" because you don't eat or drink anything other than six bottles of SueroViv each day.

Here's the recommended protocol for consuming SueroViv cultured whey beverages, whether you're on a three-day or one-day cleanse:

- 7:30 A.M.: one bottle of SueroViv or Suero Gold

- 10 A.M.: one bottle of SueroViv or Suero Gold

- 12:30 P.M.: one bottle of SueroViv or Suero Gold

- 2 P.M.: one bottle of SueroViv or Suero Gold

- 4:30 P.M.: one bottle of SueroViv or Suero Gold

- 7 P.M.: one bottle of SueroViv or Suero Gold

SueroViv contains organic, cultured whey from exclusively green-fed cattle. Some people say that after a day or two on the Suero Cleanse, they experience symptoms of detoxification such as a coated tongue or even digestive rumblings, which are common during the cleansing experience.

Cultured whey supports the body's cleansing mechanisms because it contains high-quality, structured H_2O and an excellent balance of sodium and potassium. Sodium pumps water and nutrients into the cells and potassium pumps waste products out of the cells.

With its abundance of probiotics, enzymes, and vitamins, cultured whey is an all-around health elixir and certainly hard to beat.

13

THE MEAT YOU EAT

In the first chapter of the Book of Daniel, we read:

> *Daniel then said to the guard whom the chief official had appointed over Daniel, Hananiah, Mishael and Azariah, "Please test your servants for ten days: Give us nothing but vegetables to eat and water to drink. Then compare our appearance with that of the young men who eat the royal food, and treat your servants in accordance with what you see." So he agreed to this and tested them for ten days* (Daniel 1:11-14 NIV).

This passage from Daniel is taken from the New International Version, one of a dozen translations of the Bible into modern English. Because "vegetables" is the favored present-day translation of the Hebrew word for "pulse"—a translation not quite correct, as I mentioned earlier—many people think Daniel and his friends were vegetarians.

I don't think that was the case at all.

First off, the Hebrew people weren't vegetarians 2,600 years ago. Sure, there were periods when they undoubtedly went without meat, but feasting and celebratory times always called for the "fatted calf." I'm positive that Daniel participated in the festivals prescribed in the Law of Moses, including the consumption of the Passover lamb. He had studied the Torah, which recounted meat being eaten by Abraham, Isaac, Jacob, and Moses.

Even though the science of Daniel's time hadn't identified protein—or fats or carbohydrates—they deduced that meat does a body good. Perhaps they felt healthier, stronger, or could stay on task longer after consuming meat. Whatever the reason, I believe Daniel, Hananiah, Misha-el, and Azariah loved a good New York (or Jerusalem) strip steak as much as anyone else.

But when offered a "daily amount of food and wine from the king's table," the four freshmen were resolute: they wanted to stand up for the God of heaven whom they faithfully served. I believe the reason they wanted no part of this fare was because they regarded the meats gracing the king's table as "detestable" or "unclean." I touched on this in the Introduction when I described how the Hebrew people were forbidden from consuming foods considered detestable in Leviticus 11. They were also told in explicit terms what meats they *could* eat.

God, in His infinite wisdom, didn't beat around the burning bush when He directed Moses to tell the Israelites, "Of all the animals that live on land, these are the ones you may eat: You may eat any animal that has a divided hoof and that chews the cud" (Leviticus 11:2-3 NIV). Examples of these types of animals are cows, goats, sheep, oxen, deer, buffalo, and other wild game.

Here are some other points that the Lord made in Leviticus:

- The camel, though it chewed the cud, did not have a split hoof, making it unclean to eat.

- Badgers, rabbits, and pigs fit the same description. "You must not eat their meat or touch their carcasses; they are unclean for you," the Lord said in Leviticus 11:8.

- Birds or fowl that ate flesh, such as vultures, were unclean, but birds that pecked on insects and grains for food—such as quail or doves—were clean.

- Hard-shelled crustaceans such as lobster, crabs, or clams were to be avoided, as well as some smooth-skinned species, such as catfish and eel.

- Fish that could be eaten were ones with fins and scales, such as trout, salmon, snapper, and grouper.

Of all the animals listed as detestable, pigs were probably Public Enemy Number 1 for the Hebrew people. There's something about these barnyard animals that make them inconceivable to eat for those following God's commandments. I know that's far different in our culture, where pork is marketed as the "other white meat," bacon strips are routinely laced across fast-food cheeseburgers, and pork barbecue is revered throughout the Deep South.

But let's talk about swine for a moment. (Doesn't the word *swine* sound a lot worse than *pigs*?)

These mobile trash compactors love nothing better than to stand in knee-deep muck and dip their dirty snouts into mounds of garbage and leftovers. They'll eat any swill thrown their way. Besides feasting on slop, they'll even dig into the carcasses and body parts of other pigs. I often recount the story that comes from the excellent book, *God's Key to Health and Happiness* by Rev. Elmer Josephson, about a pig farmer who stacked ten pigs in individual wire cages on top of one another. He fed the pig in the penthouse cage a normal diet and let the rest of the pigs eat the droppings from the pig above. Everyone survived just fine, except maybe those who ate the resulting pork chops!

When Daniel was being educated in the Torah, he undoubtedly learned that the Hebrew word used to describe "unclean meats" could also be translated as "detestable," "foul," "polluted," and "putrid," the same terms used to describe human waste. He understood well that God was quite serious when He directed him to keep unclean meats at arm's length.

Daniel was also quite serious about obeying God. We learn this in Daniel 1:

> *But Daniel purposed in his heart that he would not defile himself with the portion of the king's delicacies, nor with the wine which he drank; therefore he requested of the chief of the eunuchs that he might not defile himself* (Daniel 1:8).

Defile is the operative word here. No way would Daniel damage his relationship with God by eating unclean meats that he had *never* eaten before. While the Bible isn't exactly clear which meats from which animals were on the king's table that day, I believe that in addition to being "detestable," or "unclean," the king's delicacies fell into one of three biblically prohibited categories:

1. *The meats were likely ceremonially sacrificed to Babylonian idols.*

"Appeasing" the gods of Nebuchadnezzar's day meant sacrificing something of great worth. In those days, that was livestock. When meat was slaughtered on the altar of a pagan god, then it was sacrificed in that god's honor.

2. *The meats were unclean because the animals had been strangled and/ or their blood had not been drained.*

Leviticus 17 says that meat should not be eaten if the animal was not "bled out" during slaughter, which was always performed with a sharp knife that was generally twice as long as the diameter of the animal's neck. The *shochet* (the person performing the slaughter) was instructed to sever with one motion the trachea, esophagus, and blood vessels of the neck, which minimized suffering and resulted in the animal dying within seconds and then bleeding out.

Leviticus 17:11 says, "The life of the flesh is in the blood," which underscores the importance of removing as much blood as possible. Most non-kosher meat companies—even organic and grass-fed producers—slaughter cattle with trauma to the head, which may result in pooling of the blood and an increase in adrenaline, which impacts the quality of the meat.

3. *The meats were contaminated with fat.*

There are several references in Leviticus about removing all the fat around the internal organs, lungs, and kidneys before consuming the meat. The small streaks of fat found within and on the muscle—what we call "marbling" today—were okay to eat.

Was there fish served at the King's table? We don't know, but Daniel and his friends would have turned their backs on hard-shelled crustaceans such as lobster, crabs, and clams, as well as catfish and eel.

Like hogs in a pigpen, these scavengers of the oceans and lakes are bottom-feeders that troll along the seabed or lakebed, slurping up fish droppings, for lack of a better term. The good news is they purify the water; the bad news is that their diet consists of gulping you-know-what. Whatever they consume goes straight into their systems, which explains why today scientists measure pollution in the water by checking the flesh of scallops, oysters, crabs, clams, and lobsters for toxin levels—and why Daniel and his friends refused to eat these foods.

TOP SOURCES OF PROTEIN

Protein-rich foods such as meat, poultry, and fish are important to good health, which is why I do not advocate a strictly vegetarian diet. Responsible for building and repairing tissue, protein ranks as the most important nutrient that your body needs—even more important than fats and much more essential than carbohydrates. If you don't consume enough protein, your body will wither and become very weak. Protein is *that* important.

Besides driving the engine of growth and development within your body, protein accomplishes the following tasks:

- manufactures hormones, antibodies, enzymes, and tissues

- helps maintain the proper acid-alkaline balance in your body

Most muscles, organs, and hormones are comprised of protein. Since the human body simply does not store proteins for later use, as it does with carbohydrates and to a greater extent fats, you have to continually replenish the body's stores by consuming protein-rich foods.

What are the best, most "complete" sources of protein for the body? They are:

- organically raised, pasture-fed beef, lamb, goat, buffalo, and venison

- wild-caught fish with scales and fins from oceans and rivers

- pastured poultry and eggs

- cultured dairy products derived from cow's milk (free of A1 beta-casein, as you'll learn in the next chapter), goat's milk, and sheep's milk

What are the worst sources of protein that are commonly eaten today? The answer is pork and shellfish, which I urge you to strike from your diet as well as imitation meat products made from processed and often genetically modified soy.

I realize this advice will be controversial in your household, but I believe that following it will result in the betterment of your family's health. What was unclean for Daniel and his friends thousands of years ago is still unclean today.

Does that mean we're supposed to follow this advice from the Old Testament? While I agree that the atoning sacrifice of Jesus paid the price for us and we are justified by His grace, I believe it is the freedom we have in Christ that empowers us to honor His commandments. So if you're asking me, "Can I eat biblically detestable meats such as pork and shellfish and still get to heaven?" my answer is simple: "Yes, but you'll likely get there a lot sooner."

That said, I still believe God's dietary commandments from Leviticus and Deuteronomy are relevant and important to us today and should be observed for our own good.

Let me use an example to explain why. Imagine that you were invited to the biggest church potluck ever, one where the buffet table ringed the perimeter of the fellowship hall. Just about every food known has been set out—thick sirloins fresh off the barbeque, sweet corn on the cob, robust salads, and homemade desserts. At the same time, some folks brought their favorite scampi and pasta dishes, while another family went all out and brought a pot of steaming lobster. Some harried couples didn't have time to cook, so they stopped by the supermarket and purchased fried chicken and chocolate chip cookies for the dessert table.

You're free to pick and choose what you want to eat from those buffet tables; that's called God's grace. But what would be the healthiest items to put on your plate? I don't think lobster, scampi with pasta, fried chicken, and store-bought chocolate chip cookies would be the wise choices.

Where the rubber meets the road for me is that God called pork products and shellfish "unclean" and "detestable" thousands of years ago, so how has that changed? Furthermore, why would I want to introduce unclean meats into my body, which is called God's temple in I Corinthians 3:16?

"Clean," biblically correct examples of red meats would be organically raised cattle, sheep, goats, buffalo, and venison; "clean" poultry and fowl would be pasture-raised chicken and quail; and "clean" fish would be wild-caught fish such as sockeye salmon, halibut, walleye, and lake trout.

Pasture-raised beef is leaner and lower in calories than conventionally produced grain-fed beef. Pastured beef is higher in heart-friendly omega-3 fatty acids and important vitamins such as vitamins B12 and E, and, in my opinion, is much healthier for you than meat from hormone-injected cattle eating pesticide-sprayed feed laced with antibiotics. Pasture-

What If I'm a Vegetarian?

If you've made a choice to live life as a vegetarian or a vegan, I respect that decision. What vegetarians must do—especially the strict ones—is exercise constant vigilance. While nuts, seeds, legumes, cereal grains, and fermented soy products are decent protein sources, vegetarians have to be careful to give their bodies enough protein to provide essential amino acids such as methionine, cysteine, and cystine, which are crucial to the brain and nervous system. Lacto-ovo vegetarians have an easier time of it because they can consume high-quality protein sources such as eggs and cultured dairy.

The bottom line is that it's crucial for vegetarians and vegans to be proactive about what they choose to eat—and careful to consume several top-quality vegetable proteins and healthy fats from sources that include sprouted nuts and seeds, avocados, and coconut products.

fed beef is high in conjugated linoleic acid (CLA), a fatty acid that appears to modestly reduce body fat while preserving muscle tissue, according to researchers at the University of Wisconsin School of Medicine. Pasture-raised animals can have up to three to five times more CLA than grain-fed animals.

Now there's something about beef that you need to know: not all organic or grass-fed beef is the same, which is one reason I decided to create a new standard of beef called "Beyond Organic."

If you're seeking to produce beef that will receive the U.S. Department of Agriculture "organic" stamp of approval, the rules are complex. The USDA says cows on organic farms should have "access to pasture." If the weather doesn't allow that, then their diets can be made up of dried grass or hay, which is still a good food for cows.

The phrase "access to pasture" can be subject to interpretation. The rules state that cattle must be on pasture for at least 120 days a year, or four months, but that doesn't have to be continuous. The rest of the time, at least 30 percent of "dry matter" of their diet must come from grass. The other 70 percent? That can be grain-based feed.

But the real difference is how the cattle "finish" before they go the slaughter floor. In the conventional world, cattle go to the feedlot for 90 to 180 days before they're processed, where they are fed—almost exclusively—grain that's been laced with growth-promoting chemicals as well as other byproducts you don't want to hear about. This growth-spurt formula is the backbone of the U.S. beef industry and represents roughly 90 percent of all available beef produced in America. A feedlot steer can grow to slaughter weight up to a year faster than a cow fed only green forage such as grass and hay.

In the organic world, though, there's some wiggle room.

According to USDA organic standards, producers of organic beef can put their animals in "organic feedlots" for the last four months of their lives. In other words, cattle can be bunched up in pens and fed organic grain (no GMOs, hormones, or antibiotics) while they stand in one place, packing on the pounds before their date with destiny. It's anyone's guess as to how many organic beef producers are taking advantage of this rule.

At Beyond Organic, we have a different finishing program for our cattle that is, essentially, the "anti-feedlot." We start our animals and finish them on organic greens in our open pastures. During our finishing process, the cattle are offered a three-day, specially designed bovine detox program, if they need it. The bovine detox program is comprised of a combination of minerals and other compounds that help remove toxins from the body.

In addition to our unique GreenFinishing program, we employ biblical slaughter methods in our beef processing. Our processing procedures adhere to animal kindness standards developed by famed agricultural scientist Dr. Temple Grandin.

We go to all this effort so that we can produce one of the best sources of protein on the planet. Our GreenFinished Beef contains:

- vitamin E, beta-carotene, and vitamin C

- vitamin B12, iron, and zinc

- a healthy ratio of omega-6 fatty acids to omega-3 fatty acids and conjugated linoleic acid (CLA)

One of the greatest benefits of our GreenFinished Beef is its great taste, and taste is important. In fact, I've had plenty of people over the years approach me at my seminars and say, "I want to eat grass-fed beef, but it's tough and tastes like cardboard."

I understand where they are coming from, and I enjoy the taste of a good steak myself. I'm learning to appreciate real food and understand that good health is the greatest taste of all.

While I place a strong emphasis on the health benefits of the foods I consume, I must say that our Beyond Organic steaks, ranch roasts, cheddar sausage grillers, and even our BarBQ beef jerky are top notch!

GO FOR WILD-CAUGHT AND PASTURED

Let me close this chapter with a few words about the other two meats commonly consumed in American diets—fish and chicken.

There's a disturbing way that fish and chicken are raised and produced for common consumption. The "Atlantic salmon" served in restaurants and on display in supermarket cases has been grown on fish farms, where the salmon spend their days cooped up in concrete tanks, fattening up on pellets of dubious man-made chow, not streaking through the ocean gobbling up small marine life as they're supposed to. There's no way these "feedlot salmon" or farm-raised tilapia and trout measure up to their cold-water cousins in terms of taste or nutritional value.

Wild-caught fish are always going to be an absolutely incredible food and should be consumed liberally. Fish caught in the wild provide a richer source of omega-3 fats, protein, vitamins, and minerals.

As for chicken, everything can be summed by this statement: chicken is cheap, tastes good, and adapts well to sauces and spices. No wonder it's the country's most popular meat.

The Egg-ceptional Egg

I've heard the voices in the popular culture say that eggs are bad for you because they're high in cholesterol.

Don't listen to them because God created a nearly perfect protein source in the humble egg.

Within the thin shell is a nutrient-dense food that packs six grams of protein, as well as vitamin B-12, vitamin E, lutein, riboflavin, folic acid, calcium, zinc, iron, essential fatty acids, and all eight essential amino acids. All this in a nifty sixty-eight calorie package.

Pastured eggs are unsung heroes that provide outstanding nutrition and are great to add to smoothies.

It's no secret that commercial chickens are raised in horrible and inhumane conditions—stuffed into floor-to-ceiling cages inside stuffy enclosed barns. They do not go outside for the duration of their short dreary lives, and their "living space" is the size of a standard sheet of printing paper. They are raised to gain weight as quickly as possible, fed antibiotics to fend off illness, and live no more than three months before ending up in a refrigerator case.

While commercially produced chickens are raised entirely indoors with tens of thousands of other chickens in close quarters, never seeing the sun or pasture, organic or "free range" chickens may have a life only marginally better. I say that because there's no standard definition or industry guidelines on how long chickens need to be outdoors in pasture.

In addition, the USDA definition of "free-range" is in the eyes of the beholder. Some poultry producers interpret "access to pasture" as a small "doggie door" at the end of a hundred-foot shed filled with uncaged birds moving around the litter-covered floor. Many never bother to push through the door and go outside.

Others feel as though the spirit of the rules means that the birds have to get outside in the open air and sunshine, but their "free range" extends no further than a dirt patch, where some sort of feed has been set out for them to pluck on. Meanwhile, consumers have certain expectations for what a "certi-fied organic" sticker on the whole fryer packaging means, and they would be surprised to learn that their organic chicken was cooped up most of the day, pecking at grain.

So do some homework to make sure that chicken you're buying—and eggs for that matter—carry the designation "pastured." While pastured poultry and eggs are premium products carrying a hefty price tag, I believe they are worth every penny.

14

THE LAND OF MILK AND HONEY

I, like most believers in Jesus, had a longing to visit Israel. The land of the Bible, the Holy Land where Jesus walked—Israel is all of this and more.

My one and only trip to the Holy Land happened in October 1998. I was twenty-three years old and traveling on a tour organized by my home church at the time, Christ Fellowship in Palm Beach Gardens. This was a great opportunity to travel to Israel and experience the Promised Land, so I took it. Being Jewish only added to my anticipation of visiting such a historic place—which housed the roots of my past as well as the very symbol of my faith.

Joining the tour group was a young lady named Nicki Tackett, whom I had met in the singles' group that gathered on Monday nights at Christ Fellowship. We were dating at the time and both felt the desire to get married in the near future. While in Israel, I even remember shopping for a diamond in Tel Aviv. No luck on finding an affordable Israeli gemstone, but we did marry less than a year later.

Our group saw all the usual and popular historic sights. I loved Mount Carmel and the statue of Elijah reenacting the fire he called down from heaven. Seeing where Jesus spoke the Beatitudes at the Mount of Olives was awe-inspiring, as well as visiting Megiddo, the "Hill of Battles" where archeologists have uncovered twenty civilizations built upon one another.

Joining us on the trip was Hall of Fame baseball catcher Gary Carter and his wife, Sandy, which was a welcome surprise to this lifelong baseball fan. I talked Gary's ear off, bringing up every baseball stat known to man, but he was a good sport and indulged my excitement. When our discussions turned to nutrition, he was receptive to hearing my thoughts because he was having huge problems with his aching knees after many years of crouching behind the plate. (Sadly, Gary would face far more serious health problems. He died from brain cancer in 2012 at the age of fifty-seven.)

If I had to pick a few other highlights from our trip to Israel, I'd say that swimming in the Dead Sea and getting baptized in the Jordan River topped the list. It was awesome seeing the very places I had read so much about in the Bible. This was the land of "milk and honey" promised to Moses and the Hebrew people in Exodus 3:8. The Angel of the Lord said that He had seen the oppression of His people in Egypt and that He would deliver them out of the hands of their captors and lead them to a "land flowing with milk and honey."

For the Hebrew people, there was great symbolism in associating the Promised Land with foods such as milk and honey. If the land was flowing with milk, that meant their livestock would graze on wide-open fields of lush pasture, producing plentiful milk. The honey would come from bees that thrived on land blessed with a natural abundance of flowers, in addition to honey made from fruits such as dates and grapes.

It's interesting that the Bible's Promised Land was called the land of milk and honey, yet today, many nutrition experts encourage dieters to avoid dairy and sweets. I believe that milk and honey, when consumed in their correct forms, can be wonderful foods.

Unfortunately, most of the dairy and sweeteners we consume today are anything but healthy.

GOT MILK?

Nearly 800 years before His birth, the prophet Isaiah wrote 123 prophecies about the coming Messiah. Four of those prophecies are found in the seventh chapter of the Book of Isaiah:

- The Messiah would be born of a virgin (Isaiah 7:14).

- The Messiah would be called Immanuel, *God with Us* (Isaiah 7:14).

- The Messiah would be God (Isaiah 7:14).

- The Messiah would have wisdom from a young age (Isaiah 7:15).

The last bullet point refers to this verse:

Curds and honey He shall eat, that He may know to refuse the evil and choose the good (Isaiah 7:15).

A better understanding of Isaiah 7:15 comes from the original New Living Translation, printed in 1996:

By the time this child is old enough to eat curds and honey, he will know enough to choose what is right and reject what is wrong.

What Scripture is saying here is that Jesus would know right from wrong from the time He was a preschooler, when He ate His curds and honey.

Curds or cheese are made when milk is separated out into solids (curds) and liquid (whey). The white curds are slippery and have a gelatinous feel to them. Curds have a pleasant and slightly tart taste resulting from the enzymatic pre-digestion they undergo during the cheese-making process.

Back in Jesus' time, curds were very popular in the spring and fall, traditionally the times of year when the rains came and the pastures were abundant with nutrition for the cows, sheep, and goats that produced copious amounts of milk. Since there was no refrigeration, our biblical ancestors looked for ways to preserve the milk, and forming it into curds added significantly to its conservation. Honey from bees had to be a rare treat for young and old alike back in biblical times.

When it comes to dairy products and sweeteners in your daily diet, it's really important to choose wisely. I'll start first with dairy by saying that any time you talk about milk, you're sure to stir up some controversy.

There are voices who believe we shouldn't consume any milk or dairy products. They say our bodies have no need for milk after we've been weaned. Our bodies weren't designed to drink the milk of another species, they point out.

Nearly forty years ago, my parents bought in to those arguments. They were vegans when I was born, so we didn't have any milk or dairy products in our house for the first four and a half years of my life—or meat, for that matter. They had a change of heart when Mom became pregnant with my sister, Jenna. Mom began to crave the nutrients found in meat and dairy products to nourish the life growing inside her.

I think any assertions that humans shouldn't consume dairy after weaning are ridiculous. Humans have been consuming dairy for thousands of years, and our Old Testament forefathers practically lived off of the dairy produced by their flocks and herds, especially in the winter months when there were no fruit on the trees, vegetables in the garden, or grains in the field.

As for the argument that we're the only ones who drink another species' milk, I point out that if you put milk in front of another animal—for instance, cow's milk in a saucer for your dog or cat—your pet will gladly lap up that milk. To say that humans are the only ones who drink another species' milk is a silly analogy, as we're also the only ones to send text messages or Skype!

I believe the right kind of dairy is wonderful for your health. I've long championed the consumption of cultured dairy products, which are abundant in probiotics, enzymes, and easily digestible proteins.

Ever since my first book *Patient, Heal Thyself* was released in late 2002, I have recommended the consumption of dairy products made from goat's milk and sheep's milk to the exclusion of cow's milk. It always seemed to me that goat's milk and sheep's milk were easier to digest and assimilate than cow's milk, but I never really understood why.

That would start to change in 2006 when I visited Hendricks Farms and Dairy in Telford, Pennsylvania, while on a speaking tour. I immediately noted that the owner, Trent Hendricks, had a passion to raise food sustainably and locally. After my first sampling, I can attest that his award-winning raw milk cheese, eggs from pastured chickens, and meats such as lamb sausage were delicious and nutritious, which is why health-minded people would drive hundreds of miles to buy his superior grass-fed meats and dairy products.

Trent's grass-fed raw milk ice cream was otherworldly. That afternoon, I tried scoops of vanilla, maple, strawberry, and peanut butter and couldn't decide which I liked best. On a personal note, I found the Hendricks Farms' dairy products to be very easy to digest, more so than other cow's milk dairy I'd consumed in the past.

Trent and I discussed the makeup of cow's milk, which consists of fat, protein, carbohydrates, vitamins, minerals, and water. The protein is primarily made up of two proteins: the first is called casein (about 80 percent) and the other is lactalbumin or whey (the remaining 20 percent). Within the casein is a particular protein called beta-casein with two primary variations—A1 and A2—depending on the genetic makeup of the cow the milk came from.

The A1 beta-casein affects the body differently than A2 beta-casein does. Upon digestion of A1 beta-casein, a peptide—a small fragment of protein—is formed. Known as beta-casomorphin 7, or BCM7, if this peptide gets through the stomach and into the blood, it may cause the body some problems. That could explain why many people who can't tolerate cow's milk complain of bloating, cramps, gas, and diarrhea. What was previously understood to be symptoms of lactose intolerance may in fact be an intolerance to the A1 beta-casein protein.

I nodded my head while Trent expounded on the topic of dairy intolerance. From reading my books, Trent knew that I was a big proponent of milk from goats and sheep.

Trent suggested that there might be more to the story. He believed that good quality cow's milk could be tolerated just as well as milk from goats and sheep and could be even healthier, provided that the cow produced milk free of A1 beta-casein.

This was the first I heard on the subject. Could the presence of A1 beta-casein in most cow's milk—even raw, grass-fed—be the reason why many can't tolerate it?

I did my own research and found that all milk produced by goats and sheep is free of A1 beta-casein. I also learned that 99.9 percent of cow's milk in the

U.S. contains A1 beta-casein. But outside the United States, cows in Africa, India, and the Middle East produced milk that was free of A1 beta-casein due to the fact that their cattle originated from a different species.

Why did some cows have A1 beta-casein and others didn't? It's believed that a biological mutation that occurred hundreds, if not thousands, of years ago created a new subspecies of cow, known as *bos taurus*, with the genetics to produce an aberrant protein in its milk. These *bos taurus* cows became the dominant species of cattle in Europe, the United States, as well as in New Zealand and Australia.

On the other hand, *bos indicus* cattle (also known as Zebu) originated in the subcontinent of India and became the dominant species of cattle in Africa and the Middle East. These cows did *not* have the genetics to produce the A1 beta-casein protein, and thus were not linked to a host of maladies.

I was intrigued by these *bos indicus* cattle without the genetics to produce A1 beta-casein and wanted to learn more.

THE RISE OF AMASAI

A few months after visiting with Trent Hendricks in Pennsylvania, Nicki and I took another trip together—this time to South Africa. I had been asked to speak at two conferences in Johannesburg.

I was poking around some grocery stores when I saw something in the dairy case called *maas*. I was told that *maas* was a traditional food inspired by the famed Maasai tribe that inhabited Tanzania and Kenya.

Maas was widely consumed in South Africa, and its preparation has been handed down generation after generation. The traditional method to make it was to start with a calabash, or a dried gourd from a tree. You drop a few cups of rice or corn with hot water into the calabash and shake it around to remove all the loose seeds. Then you rinse out the gourd a few more times.

Next, you pour in fresh milk and allow the dairy to "improve" or culture for about three days, depending on the temperature and the taste you want. The first batch will probably not taste good and will need to be thrown out until the calabash is seasoned.

The next time around, when the *maas* is ready, you pour out two-thirds and refill the gourd with more milk. You leave everything to ferment for hours or even days until it's ready.

I really liked the *maas* I tried in South Africa and felt that its unique fermentation process that infused powerful probiotics and enzymes into the milk made it superior to the popular fermented dairy products yogurt and kefir. I wondered if there was some way to replicate or produce a cultured dairy product like *maas* in the United States.

In studying the Maasai, I learned that they were a dominant tribe known for their feats of speed and strength. In fact, as a rite of passage, a Maasai teen or young man would undergo a painful circumcision and then be required to go off in the woods and kill a lion with an instrument he made by hand. Only then could he become a Maasai warrior.

The Maasai consumed a diet that was over 90 percent dairy. But not just any dairy because the cows producing milk for the Maasai were of the *bos indicus* (zebu) species that produced milk free of A1 beta-casein.

This was all starting to fit together nicely, just like a puzzle. I now understood why Africans, Arabs, Jews, and Indians who emigrated to the U.S. have such problems tolerating our country's typical dairy products. These people groups thrived on dairy from *bos indicus* (zebu) cattle free of A1 beta-casein in their homelands, but when they came to America and began consuming dairy containing A1 beta-casein, they experienced challenges.

After I purchased our land in southern Missouri and started Beyond Organic, I asked Trent Hendricks and his wife, Rachel, to lead our farming and ranching operations as well as dairy and beef production. Our first order of business was to create a beverage that would become the next generation of cultured dairy. We set out to replicate the legendary beverage of the Maasai tribe and bring it to America for the first time. By using cattle with the very same dairy-producing genetics of the Maasai, we created what I believe to be the most amazing cultured dairy beverage available today. Fittingly, and in homage to the warriors from Africa, we call it Amasai.

Amasai contains a unique balance of proteins in a complex that we call the "Z protein." The Z comes from *zebu*, which is another name for *bos indicus* cattle, otherwise known as the "original cow." Our Beyond Organic cattle have, in many ways, the same genetic makeup for milk production—or genotype—as the African cattle herded and milked by the Maasai tribe and the cattle found in India, for that matter. These types of cattle were likely milked by our biblical ancestors Abraham, Isaac, and Jacob.

Cattle from the *bos indicus* species have adapted to the hotter climates in Africa, India, and the Middle East. They have humps on the shoulders, large dewlaps, and droopy ears. They produce milk containing the Z protein complex that I believe is easily digestible and provides great benefits to people of all ages.

On the other hand, *bos taurus* cows that produce A1 beta-casein milk in the United States and in Western civilizations may be one of the reasons why so many individuals have problems digesting and tolerating milk, but hardly anyone is talking about it.

My eyes were really opened on this subject of A1 beta-casein after reading *The Devil in the Milk* by Keith Woodford, Ph.D., a professor of farm management and agribusiness at Lincoln University in New Zealand. Dr. Woodford wrote *The Devil in the Milk* a few years ago to answer the following question: *Why do health problems persist when children and adults drink commercial milk?*

Dr. Woodford was prompted to find an answer after reading about research conducted at Auckland University showing that Samoan children living in New Zealand had a much higher incidence of Type 1 diabetes than Samoan children living in Samoa. There had to be an environmental reason, not a genetic one, because the children were the same ethnicity. The only difference between the Samoa kids in New Zealand and Samoa was the milk they drank.

The devil lurking in the milk, Woodford wrote, is the BCM7 that I described earlier. The BCM7 peptide produced in the body from A1 beta-casein consumption may be even more harmful to the body than gluten, the sticky protein found in the cereal grains, wheat, rye, and barley. While gluten effects two receptor sites in the gut, affecting the body's neurological, immunological, and gastrointestinal systems, BCM7 can affect up to twenty-six receptor sites, making it potentially over ten times more dangerous than gluten.

The body recognizes BCM7 as a foreign protein and launches an attack by the immune system. If you've ever wondered why you feel increased phlegm in your lungs or digestive tract after consuming a dairy product, it could be the presence of BCM7, which selectively binds to the epithelial cells in mucous membranes and stimulates mucus production.

Dr. Woodford, in his book, makes a strong case implicating BCM7 to many serious health problems, including:

- Type 1 diabetes

- neurological impairment, including autism and schizophrenia

- impaired immune function

- autoimmune diseases

- heart disease

Depending on the genetic makeup of the person, the body can become susceptible to these sorts of illnesses as well as joint and muscle pains, fatigue, digestive disturbances, and headaches.

I urge you to check out what Dr. Woodford has to say in *The Devil in the Milk* and go online to investigate the potential dangers of A1 beta-casein for yourself. Look for sources of dairy products that do not contain A1 beta-casein as even most of the raw, grass-fed milk in America includes this potentially damaging protein. If you purchase dairy from a local farmer—which I've done in the past—then ask him (or her) if his dairy products come from milk with A1 beta-casein. If he says he's not sure, then you can be certain that his milk and cheese contain A1 beta-casein.

Don't bother researching soy milk. Most soy protein comes from genetically modified soybeans, which must be processed at high temperatures to reduce phytic acid levels. Even if the soy milk is organic, it can still cause a host of health challenges affecting the digestive and endocrine systems. Store-bought rice milk and almond milk are a bit better than soy, but what you're really getting is a beverage that's been highly processed. Making your own raw almond milk can be very healthy, if you're willing to invest the time.

Because of what I've learned about A1 beta-casein in the last few years, the Rubin family has made it a point not to consume dairy products containing this protein. Not only does my family consume our cultured dairy beverage Amasai, but we also eat liberally from our collection of Beyond Organic GreenFed raw cheeses. I'm proud to say that all of the dairy products coming from our Beyond Organic ranches in southern Missouri are made from cows free of the A1 beta-casein gene. Few, if any, dairy operations in the United States can make this claim.

Nicki and I tease each other regarding whether we view our cheeses as delicacies or nutritional powerhouses. I think they're both. Beyond Organic cheeses come from dairy cows on our GreenFed program, which means they graze to their hearts' content on a "salad bar" of grasses, legumes, herbs, and forbs found in our pastures.

Our cheeses are incredible taste sensations, including our pungent Beyond Organic Danish Sky (blue-style cheese) and our creamy and smooth Beyond Organic Alpine White (Brie-style cheese). These cheeses are also power-houses of predigested protein and healthy fats including omega-3 fatty acids and CLA—conjugated linoleic acid—plus much-needed probiotics, key minerals, and a vitamin known as K_2. In fact, cheese, particularly soft brie-style cheese, is the richest source of vitamin K_2 in the American diet.

Vitamin K_2 is a star-studded fat-soluble vitamin that produces a protein called osteocalcin, which assists the body in the incorporation of calcium into the bones, a process vital for bone growth and bone metabolism. I believe vitamin K_2 is the second most important vitamin after vitamin D, which is critical for building strong, healthy bones and is also required for the body to absorb calcium.

Dr. Weston A. Price, a health pioneer and a nutritional hero of mine, referred to vitamin K_2 as "Activator X" because of the fundamental role this nutrient plays in helping the body facilitate the absorption of minerals to build healthy bones in children and to promote a strong, healthy skeletal system for people entering middle age and the senior years.

The only better known dietary source for vitamin K_2 is a Southeast Asian condiment known as natto, which is made from fermented boiled soybeans.

The sticking point with most Americans is natto's taste and aroma. There's no doubt that natto's stinky smell can be a stumbling block, which is why natto is best eaten when served over rice. Many claim it's better tasting than its Limburger cheese-like smell indicates.

Our Beyond Organic cheeses smell good and are really raw, with milk temperatures never exceeding a cow's body temperature of 101.5, making this delicious treat a source of live enzymes and probiotics. Many raw cheeses heat their milk to temperatures as high as 144 degrees, which can damage the integrity of the product.

If you're wondering what makes our dairy truly Beyond Organic, here are some reasons:

1.   **Z milk.** Producing milk with a unique and beneficial balance of proteins to provide health to people of all ages is a priority.

2.   **GreenFed.** Beyond Organic cattle consume only green foods such as grasses, herbs, forbs, and legumes. Our goal is to be completely sustainable, producing all of the feed our cattle need in the form of organic nutrient-dense pastures. Blades of grass can be compared to tiny solar panels, capturing the power of the sun and transferring that energy to the cattle and then to us in the form of cheese and cultured dairy products. Most organic dairies feed grain to their cattle, and that alters the fatty acids in the milk.

3.   **Natural breeding.** Most organic and conventional dairies utilize artificial insemination to breed their cows. Beyond Organic's breeding strategy includes the use of specially selected bulls with the Zebu genetic, which can create healthy and hardy cattle that are extremely adaptable to our climate and environment with great longevity. Selecting the right bulls is a key to transforming any cow herd.

4.   **Natural calf rearing.** Every conventional dairy and most organic dairies I know of pull the calf from the mom immediately after birth; the calf is fed formula and supplemented with pellets while spending the first three to six months of life in a small crate. At Beyond Organic farms and ranches, we have conducted research on the difference in health and maturation of calves raised naturally in groups fed raw milk from our herd versus calves raised by momma cows. The staggering results have caused us to implement a natural

calf-rearing strategy with momma-raised calves exhibiting far greater health, growth, and maturity than those raised in calf groups without momma cows. While this requires us to keep a 25 percent to 50 percent larger herd, the health of our cows is definitely worth it.

5.   Once-a-day milking. Modern dairies milk cattle two to six times per day, minimizing the amount of time the cows can spend soaking up the sun on green pastures. The Beyond Organic way is to milk cows once per day, allowing them to spend more than twenty-three hours per day outdoors on pasture where they belong.

6.   Seasonal dairy. Harkening back to dairying practices of old, Beyond Organic employs a seasonal dairy strategy, allowing our cattle and our pastures to rest and recuperate during periods of challenging weather.

7.   Vaccination free. To my surprise, organic standards allow for vaccinations of cattle. Our goal is to raise a healthy herd with natural immunity.

8.   Animal kindness. We practice humane animal standards at Beyond Organic. We allow calves to stay with their mothers and cultivate in an environment where our cattle can live long and productive lives.

9.   Olde World production methods. Beyond Organic dairy is highly nutritious, and to maintain that value, it's critical to use the gentlest form of processing. The milk used for our cultured dairy beverage Amasai is processed slowly and gently, taking up to 180 times longer than other organic dairy. Our cheese making is accomplished with extreme care in order to maintain the "live food" quality of our raw milk.

10.   Farmstead. We believe that the best dairy is produced on the same farm that the cows are born and raised. Most dairy production is centralized today with milk traveling hundreds of miles from farm to processor. At Beyond Organic, we produce our dairy products immediately after milking, all on the same farm.

11.   Artisanal. Creating healthy and delicious cheeses and cultured dairy products is a combination of art and science. In my opinion, the only way to ensure the highest quality is to produce these products in small batches the Beyond Organic way.

12. **Probiotic infused.** Probiotic means "for life," and all Beyond Organic dairy products are infused with powerful probiotics to support healthy digestion and immune system function.

Following all these measures has a cost: at Beyond Organic, we estimate that we produce 60 percent less milk than organic cows fed a high-grain diet. But the milk coming out of our cows to produce Amasai and our really raw green-fed cheeses makes the effort well worth the investment.

I've already told you about Amasai, so now let me describe our Beyond Organic cheeses in greater detail:

🧀 **Beyond Organic Raw Cheddar Reserve** is made from our spring or fall milk and thus has a limited production run. The cheese is aged for a minimum of nine months to carry the "reserve" title. Our cheddar cheese is mature and characterized by its sharp cheddar taste.

🧀 **Beyond Organic Raw Havarti Reserve** is creamy and smooth but with a bold taste slightly milder than our Cheddar Reserve.

🧀 **Beyond Organic Danish Sky** is creamy with pungent blue cheese overtones. I grew up narrow in my food choices and wouldn't try blue cheese as a child. It wasn't until Nicki opened up my eyes to the delights of the culinary world that I finally sampled blue cheese—and loved it. Highly nutritious and loaded with beneficial compounds, Danish Sky is great on top of steaks off the grill. Or you can combine our blue style cheese with Amasai in a blender to make the best-tasting blue cheese dressing ever. Pass the lettuce wedge, please.

🧀 **Beyond Organic Alpine White** is a subtle, brie style creamy cheese that is easily spreadable and best eaten when gooey. This delicious soft cheese is a taste treat when spread on our EA Live Seven Seed Crackers. Like Danish Sky, our Alpine White comes in 12-ounce mini wheels. Watch out—you might eat an entire wheel in one sitting. That's what Nicki did when she came upon a particularly yummy batch.

🧀 **Beyond Organic Jack Cheese** is a favorite for adults and children alike. This adaptable cheese is great on sandwiches and in salads.

🧀 **Beyond Organic Raw Cheddar Bites** could be the most unique cheese in America. It's certainly a solution to the raw milk dilemma.

To make our Raw Cheddar Bites, we take our raw milk and separate it into curds and whey—the start of the cheese-making process. The raw milk curds are allowed to age for sixty days, which is the minimum amount of time a raw cheese must be aged. The resulting cheese is similar to string cheese, with a soft, creamy texture and clean flavor.

Don't Look to Goat's Milk or Sheep's Milk as Your First Choice

There's a good news/bad news situation with goat's milk and sheep's milk.

The good news first: goats and sheep produce milk free of A1 beta-casein. That means their milk doesn't create the BCM7 peptide when ingested, which seems to cause so many issues with people.

The bad news? Besides the perceived negative taste with goat's milk, there aren't any readily available organic brands of goat's milk that I'm aware of. Because goats don't exclusively graze and prefer to browse, almost every goat farm that I've seen or observed has them eating large amounts of grains, which affects the fatty acid composition of the milk. In addition, goats have issues with parasites and, therefore, are often de-wormed.

The same goes for sheep's milk. You can't find any organic dairy products made from sheep's milk in stores these days, which probably has to do with the medical treatments they require. The other problem is that sheep's milk products are in short supply.

Talk about concentrated raw milk protein. For every ounce of Raw Cheddar Bites, you receive the same quantity of protein and healthy fats as one glass of raw milk. The Raw Cheddar Bites come in a pouch and can be eaten by hand, mixed into a salad, or placed on a sprouted seed cracker.

All of our Beyond Organic raw cheeses provide the goodness of raw milk to people all over America. Despite its great health benefits, raw dairy products can be legally sold in only a handful of states, with the regulators cracking down more and more with each passing year. I believe raw milk is ideal, but finding safe, reliable sources is difficult in the best of circumstances. Our Beyond Organic raw cheeses are safe, nutritious, and incredibly tasty.

So if you've sworn off raw dairy because it's not readily available or a hassle to find—or if you've sworn off dairy because your stomach doesn't tolerate A1 beta-casein very well, then give our Beyond Organic dairy with Z protein a try.

Many have commented to me that Beyond Organic has healed their relationship with dairy. All I can say is, "Well put."

MAKE IT SHORT AND SWEET

As for the sweet side of the "land of milk and honey," my favorite sweetener is raw honey, a superfood from the hive. Raw, unheated honey is the original sweetener and was extolled by the wisest man who ever lived—Solomon—in a personal, intimate way. "My son, eat honey because it is good, and the honeycomb which is sweet to your taste" (Proverb 24:13).

Honey has been around for thousands of years, long before humankind knew about all the antioxidants, enzymes, vitamins, and minerals within the thick, golden nectar produced by bees. Raw honey is superb to sweeten smoothies, Amasai, tea, and a zillion other foods.

Evaporated coconut nectar has become another sweet favorite of mine. Also known as coconut sugar, this type of sweetener is not made from coconut meat but from tapping the coconut tree and draining the sap in a process similar to producing maple syrup from a maple tree. Coconut sugar is naturally low on the glycemic index scale, which is a plus. Here's an interesting bit of trivia: when a coconut palm tree is tapped for its sap, the tree can no longer grow coconuts.

Even though maple syrup is heated during the production, I'm fine with this natural sugar, as long as it is whole organic maple syrup. What I'm not so excited about is the agave nectar that you see sold in warehouse clubs and supermarkets. Agave nectar is high in fructose and indigestible oligosaccharides, which makes it hard on the liver and difficult to digest for some people.

Sugar alcohols such as xylitol, maltitol, sorbitol, and erythritol are now routinely used in chewing gum, candy, fruit spreads, and even toothpaste and cough syrup found in health food stores. Sure, sugar alcohols taste like sugar, but the body doesn't break down or absorb sugar alcohols, which is why they are zero or low calorie. They also seem to have a laxative effect on the body.

There's another no-calorie sweetener that I'm not doing cartwheels over, and that's stevia. It's not that stevia is horrible for you by any means, but it's my belief that when you eat something sweet in nature, then the body expects energy in the form of sugars. When consuming calorie-free sweeteners, the body isn't fooled and will make up the calories somewhere else. There is a raw, whole form of stevia that is basically made from dried and ground green stevia leaves. This form of stevia is much better than the highly processed and extracted white stevia widely available.

I'm figuring that you don't need to hear a long-winded speech from me about the dangers of highly processed white granulated sugar, which is found in nearly every human-made food, from ketchup to peanut butter to teriyaki sauce. This sugar comes from sugarcane, which is then processed 99.9 percent. Besides affecting your teeth in a negative way, the heavy consumption of white sugar—along with perhaps an even more dangerous sweetener, high fructose corn syrup—is a major reason why we have a huge obesity problem in this country. All those empty calories arrive with no nutritional value while robbing the body of minerals and energy.

If you're looking for a substitute for the ubiquitous white sugar, then whole organic cane sugar is acceptable. This unrefined sugar retains many of the nutrients present in cane juice and contains amino acids, minerals, and vitamins, while table sugar is just sucrose and calories, plus traces of chemicals used in the refining process. Careful, though: even "healthier" sources of sugars must be consumed within healthy limits.

Finally, let me say a few words about artificial sweeteners—those blue, pink, and yellow packets found on restaurant tables. Researchers at Purdue University say that these sugar substitutes can interfere with the body's natural ability to count calories based on a food's sweetness. In other words, drinking an ice tea with an artificial sweetener instead of two heaping teaspoons of white sugar will reduce your caloric intake, but it could also trick the body into thinking that other sweet items don't have as many calories either.

Besides, artificial sweeteners such as aspartame, saccharin, and sucralose have sparked debate for decades because they can be highly addictive and can trigger toxic substances to cross the blood-brain barrier, causing neurological problems.

15

SUP ON SOUP

Have you ever thought about how people cooked long before we had fancy kitchens with stainless steel ovens, four-burner cooktops, and outdoor barbecue islands?

I'm talking about biblical times, when clans and families roamed as nomads, tending to their flocks, or settled in walled cities with thatched roofs over their heads. Open fires—outside the tent or inside a courtyard—served a dual purpose: they kept folks warm and provided a means of cooking. For the latter activity, they usually rigged poles to hang a heavy bronze pot over a robust fire.

Back then, the main meals of the day—served afternoon and early evening—came out of that large pot. Cooking often meant tossing a slab of boned-in meat or a whole fish into a pot or kettle and adding green vegetables, legumes, herbs, and whatever else was available. This main dish stew simmered for hours, perhaps overnight, before it was ready to be served. The everything-cooked-in-one-pot-cuisine was eaten over and over until nothing was left. Families often ate the same meal for days.

Cooking pots played a supporting role in everyday life and were referred to often in the Old Testament. Here are a few examples:

- Cooking pots are first mentioned in Exodus when the whole community of Israel grumbled about Moses and Aaron while they wandered in the wilderness. They complained that back in Egypt, "we sat around pots filled with meat and ate all the bread we wanted" (Exodus 16:3 NLT).

- In Leviticus, where the Hebrew nation was told which meats were clean and which were "detestable," they were directed to boil sacrificial meat in bronze pots and then thoroughly scour and rinse those pots (Leviticus 6:28).

- The prophet Ezekiel prophesied that Jaazaniah and Pelatiah were planning evil and giving wicked counsel in Jerusalem. In Ezekiel 11, the two men told the people in Jerusalem that they were like an iron pot. The people would be "safe as meat inside the pot," but the Lord said, "This city is an iron pot all right, but the pieces of meat are the victims of your injustice" (Ezekiel 11:7 NLT).

Stocks, bone broths, and soups have been used by ancient cultures for health purposes throughout the ages. Today, we just don't consume these nourishing foods very often, if at all, but we should. I think making one-pot meals or fresh soups using a homemade stock or broth would be a wonderful way to go back to the future.

These meals are incredibly cleansing *and* building and will change your thinking about what constitutes a dinner meal, which in most households is traditionally a slice of meat, a side of starch, and hopefully a serving of veggies. I urge you to be intentional about preparing and consuming one-pot meals and hearty soups made with real old-fashioned stock. Preparing these types of meals is a lost art these days, but with a little forethought, you can serve one of the most satisfying meals there is. On a cold winter's evening— or any other season of the year, for that matter—there's nothing better than a bowl of homemade soup.

I've sung the praises of homemade chicken soup in my previous books, but I have to say that the idea of cooking soups and meals in a single pot is a part of my family's history, as evidenced by my Grandmother Rose. You see, my grandmother grew up in a pastoral Polish village in the 1920s, the youngest of seven children born to Gidalia and Simma Katz. Even though her father owned a mill that pressed poppy seeds and flaxseeds into oil, they were considered poor, certainly by today's standards. On many occasions, there wasn't much to eat.

Here's how her parents fed a family of nine during hard times. It all began when one of them would go to the backyard chicken coop and wring a hen's neck. After plucking the feathers, the chicken would be placed in a massive cast-iron pot filled with water. A fire brought the pot to a boil and was allowed to simmer overnight. The next day, young Rose and her siblings dipped cakes of pressed flaxseeds and poppy seeds into the rendered fat that rose to the top, which was known by the Yiddish name as *schmaltz*. When food was scarce, this was a tasty treat.

After the *schmaltz* was skimmed off, the stock—which included the meat, bones, and cartilage—was used to feed her large family for an entire week—all from one chicken! What nine Katz family members received was a week's worth of extremely nutritious meals loaded with minerals, collagen, cartilage, and electrolytes. They also received generous amounts of natural gelatin, an odorless, tasteless substance that was extracted from the bones and animal tissues during the boiling process.

Everything for Grandma Rose and her family started with the stock, a liquid made from simmering meat scraps and bones.

THE MAKING OF STOCK

Today, no self-respecting chef would consider making one of his signature dishes without having stock on hand. Auguste Escoffier, considered the father of modern French classical cooking, once said, "Indeed, stock is everything in cooking...without it nothing can be done."

You don't have to be a French-trained chef to make a great stock, but you should use the bones of organic, pasture-raised cattle, lamb, or bison, pasture-raised chickens, or wild-caught fish. Stock or bone broth begins with rinsing the bones in cold water and then dropping them into a heavy-bottomed stockpot. Water is added to cover the bones, and everything is brought to a boil. Then the heat is reduced to a simmer for a minimum of twelve hours and as long as seventy-two hours. As evaporation takes its toll, you may add water once or twice during the cooking process to sufficiently cover the bones. Any layer on the surface of the water is to be skimmed off.

If you desire to make a more robust stock and to embellish upon the aforementioned bone broth, you may add to the bones a combination of vegetables (chopped carrots, celery, onion, etc.) as well as herbs, which is to be simmered along with the meaty bones. Any impurities that rise to the surface can be skimmed. You would then strain out the bones and residual veggies and have an amazing elixir that you can consume warm or use as a base for soups, grains, etc. I often recommend to people with very compromised digestion go on a broth or stock fast for a number of days to settle their system.

The best bones for making stock are cattle bones with a lot of cartilage and marrow, such as the so-called "knuckle bones" found in the various leg joints. Making stock from chicken or fish can start with a whole chicken or fish, but a great stock can be made just from the bones.

Starting with cold water seems to extract more collagen from the bones, which produces a stock with more body. You don't want to continuously boil the bones. After the initial boiling, set the stove on simmer. There's no need to stir the bones. Just be sure to keep skimming the layer off the top and to keep adding water when needed.

The essential qualities of stock—its aroma, richness, as well as many of its health-giving properties—come from the marrow of the bones. Marrow is the spongy matter inside the hard calcified matrix of the bones, from which arises blood and bone cells as well as the connective tissues—collagen—that hold your bones together. The connective tissue or collagen breaks down to form the gelatin that gives the stock body and staying power. You know you have a good stock when upon refrigeration, the appearance is a very thick gelatinous substance that is in a single, wonderful blob.

The bones used to make stock determine the kind of stock that will be produced:

- Brown stock comes from beef or veal bones, and some prefer to brown the bones in an oven before dropping them into the pot.

- Chicken stock, as you would surmise, is made from chicken bones or typically whole chickens.

- Fish stock is made from fish bones and trimmings left over after filleting.

- White stock is made from a combination of beef and chicken bones.

I would imagine that you're looking at this list and saying, I can do that. All I have to do get some leftover bones from the butcher.

Not so fast. Just as it's important and much healthier to eat pasture-fed beef, bison, or lamb, it's just as essential to use the bones from quality organic, pasture-raised sources to make your stock. Otherwise, you're taking two steps forward and one step backward in your march toward a healthier lifestyle.

You may be shocked to hear this, but it's hard to find bones from pasture-raised organic cattle this days. There must be some good word-of-mouth going around about the health properties of stocks and soups to drive up demand; either that, or there are a lot of bone broth cleansing fasts going on. If you stroll into a large health food grocery store, you're likely not to find any bones in the meat department. They often sell out the day they come in, even though they can be a bit pricey. It's not unusual to pay $20 for a three-pound package of bones from organic, grass-fed sources.

Based on the tremendous demand, we have decided to offer bones from our Beyond Organic beef and to create a delicious and nutritious bone broth so that folks all across the U.S. can enjoy the many benefits. There has been many a day when I have consumed warm or room-temperature strained beef bone broth or stock out of a tall glass before each meal. I love it so much that I often consume a pint at a time. Upon consuming, I immediately feel great.

The nutritional advantages of bone broth and stock—from calcium to phosphorus to collagen to magnesium—are noteworthy. We don't have

Beyond Organic beef stock available year round, and when we do offer it, we sell out quickly.

One area where you'll always find a good supply of stock bones is with chickens. Use the entire bird to make a delicious and nutritious chicken soup. The recuperative effects of chicken soup date as far back as the 12th century when the Jewish physician and philosopher Moses Maimonides recommended its use to improve respiratory health. In our family, homemade chicken soup was known as "Jewish penicillin," a testament to how chicken soup acts to support healthy inflammation.

Stephen Rennard, M.D., chief of pulmonary medicine at the University of Nebraska Medical Center in Omaha, Nebraska, conducted a full-blown study on the health-promoting qualities of chicken soup. He had his wife prepared a batch using a recipe from her Lithuanian grandmother. Then Dr. Rennard carted the homemade chicken soup to his laboratory, where he combined some of the soup with neutrophils to see what would happen. Neutrophils are a type of white blood cells that rush to attack an invader, which can cause fluid buildup in the pulmonary region.

As Dr. Rennard suspected, his wife's homemade chicken soup demonstrated that neutrophils showed less of a tendency to congregate, but at the same time, these neutrophils did not lose any of their ability to fight off toxins. His findings were published in *CHEST*, the peer-reviewed journal of the American College of Chest Physicians.

I'm glad that modern science is catching up to the news that chicken soup is good for the soul. Grandma Rose passed the best recipe for chicken soup on to me, a recipe based, no doubt, on the chicken soup that fueled her family in Poland in the dark days of near famine. I still haven't forgotten how she made chicken soup every few days and fed it to me when, at age twenty, I was bedridden with my health challenges.

That's why I'm sharing a new twist on my Grandma Rose's Chicken Soup recipe here, which includes directions. All you need are the right ingredients and a large stainless steel pot. One thing that Grandma Rose always added to her chicken soup recipe was cayenne pepper, which she said would clear the sinuses. I have also added the powerful spice turmeric to enhance the health benefits.

HEALING CHICKEN SOUP

Ingredients

1 whole chicken (free range, pastured, or organic chicken)	1 pound green beans
3 to 4 quarts filtered water	4 tablespoons of extra-virgin coconut oil
1 tablespoon raw apple cider vinegar or Terrain Living herbal of choice	1 bunch parsley
4 medium-sized onions, coarsely chopped	1 cup fresh or frozen green peas
8 carrots, peeled and coarsely chopped	5 garlic cloves
6 celery stalks, coarsely chopped	2 inches grated ginger
2 to 4 zucchinis, chopped	2 inches grated turmeric
	2 to 4 tablespoons of high mineral sea salt
	¼ teaspoon cayenne pepper (optional)

Directions

If you are using a whole chicken, remove giblets, neck, and any loose fat from the cavity. Place chicken or chicken pieces and chicken feet (optional) in a large stainless steel pot.

Next, add vinegar or the Terrain Living Herbal of your choice and all vegetables except parsley. Bring to a boil and simmer for 12 to 24 hours. The longer you cook the stock, the healthier the stock will be. About 30 minutes before turning off the stove, add parsley. This will impart additional mineral ions to the broth. Remove the parsley. Remove the chicken and de-bone, discard, or compost the bones. Add back the meat. Serve warm and refrigerate remaining soup once it reaches just above room temperature.

Grandma Rose's chicken soup is highly recommended during the winter to support the body's immune system and to support healthy inflammation levels. The high-fiber vegetables and healthy broth are wonderful for cleansing the body's digestive system and delicious to eat as well, especially when freezing temperatures and gray skies are the norm.

Keep in mind that stocks, broths, and bone soups are to joints and inflammation what fermented foods are to gut health. Meat stocks and bone broths promote a healthy inflammation response as well as joint health and flexibility because these meat stocks contain protein, minerals, gelatin, and fiber in a form that's easy for the body to assimilate. Gelatin from cartilage and marrow is the superstar compound, containing half of the essential amino acids we need for survival. One of those amino acids is glycine, which is needed by the liver to remove toxins from our system. Another amino acid, lysine, helps the body to absorb calcium and to build muscle.

The reason gelatin has unique powers is because of the way it attracts liquid molecules to it, which makes the digestion of cooked food easier. It's the same principle with raw foods, which contain hydrophilic colloids that attract water. Similarly, when cooked foods are served with gelatin—homemade chicken soup, for instance—the gelatin naturally binds to water and helps the food move through the digestive tract efficiently.

Gelatin also has what is called a protein-sparing effect. What protein-sparing means is that even though there might be only a gram or less of protein in a serving of strained bone broth or soup, for example, the body reacts like it received far more protein. Protein-sparing means your muscles are not wasting away but rather remain intact and strong.

The last point I want to make about broths, soups, and stocks is that besides conferring many health benefits, they also immeasurably add to the flavor of food. The rich sauces and exquisite cuisine you experience in expensive French restaurants begin with pots of stock simmering on the back burners in the restaurant kitchen. When classically trained chefs take a few ladles of this stock and put them into a saucepan, add wine and herbs and turn up the heat, they are making a reduction sauce to flavor your entrée or side dish. The good news is that the effects of the gelatin and the flavors become even *more* concentrated during the reduction process.

Yes, it takes time and forethought to prepare stocks and to make homemade stews, soups, and reduction sauces, but just think of the innumerable health benefits you and your family will receive.

You'll also go up several notches in your culinary skills!

16

FEED YOUR SKIN

During the spring of 2013, Daniel, the beloved biblical character and captive from Judah, played a supporting role in *The Bible* miniseries that ran on the History Channel for five Sundays before finishing on Easter.

I didn't get to see every episode of the biggest cable television hit of the year, but I was intrigued at how Daniel would be portrayed. The producers of *The Bible* didn't pick up Daniel's story until he was older—in his twenties—when he was part of the palace court and asked by King Nebuchadnezzar to interpret one of his dreams.

The actor who portrayed Daniel was a Swiss named Jake Canuso, so his slight Swiss-German accent was interesting. The role Canuso played did not require a lot of makeup, unlike the male actors who depicted Pharaoh and his minions, walking around marbled alcoves with shaved heads, over-the-top black eyeliner, and painted eyebrows. The royal women were heavily made up and dressed to the hilt as well. Based on the traditions of that time period, these Egyptian women likely used extensive cosmetics such as lotions and perfumes.

So, did people back in the time of Moses and Daniel really use cosmetics such as makeup, lotions, and fragrances on their bodies?

The answer is undoubtedly yes, although I doubt they had SPF 30 sunscreen at the time. What they did have were ointments, essential oil blends (known at the time as perfumes or fragrances), and individual oils or resins such as frankincense, myrrh, and aloes (sandalwood).

The first mention of essential oils, perfumes, and fragrances in the Bible occurs in Exodus 30, when the Lord instructs Moses to take quality spices such as myrrh, cinnamon, sweet-smelling cane, and cassia, and mix them with olive oil to make "an ointment compounded according to the art of the perfumer. It shall be a holy anointing oil" (Exodus 30:25).

People in biblical times availed themselves of anointing oils, lotions, and what they would call "perfumes" regularly. David, after being confronted by the prophet Nathan regarding his sin with Bathsheba—the affair that left her pregnant, which led to David's subsequent decision to have her husband, Uriah, killed on the field of battle—was told by Nathan that his infant child would die. Scripture says that David did not eat for an entire week, laying all night on the ground and pleading with the Lord for his son's life. When the boy died, however, "David arose from the ground, washed and anointed himself, and changed his clothes" (2 Samuel 12:20).

Perhaps the best example of someone using lotions, essential oils, and perfumes for skin care comes from Esther, who was part of the harem belonging King Xerxes. Esther, hoping to be selected as the new queen, followed the prescribed twelve months of beauty treatments—six months with oil of myrrh, followed by six months with special perfumes and ointments. Even thousands of years ago, women used skin and body care products for beauty.

These days, however, undergoing twelve months of intensive beauty treatments would not be a very safe thing to do. I say that because of the massive amount of chemicals found in nearly every skin and body care product on display at your neighborhood pharmacy or local supermarket.

Two of the most egregious examples are phthalates (pronounced *THA-lates*) and volatile organic compounds, or VOCs. These toxic chemicals, used to lengthen the shelf life of cosmetics, hair spray, mousses, and fragrances, are also present in perfumes, aftershave lotions, and other toiletries. And that's just the short list. You'll also find these common petroleum-based chemicals in multiplied thousands of household products such as household cleaners, furniture polishes, air fresheners, adhesives, and plastics.

The toxins present in these products enter our bodies through our skin and nasal passageway and produce a chemical residue buildup known as the *total body burden*. Although our bodies were designed to eliminate these toxins, our immune systems can overload to the point where these fat-soluble chemicals are stored in our fatty tissues, where it takes months or even years for these toxins to be eliminated—if they're eliminated at all.

When these toxins hang around, your health takes a major hit. I received a grim reminder of that recently when a fifty-seven-year-old woman diagnosed with cancer told me she believed the disease may have been caused by an accumulation of toxins in her body. Could she take back forty-four years of putting all the mascara, makeup, creams, and lotions on her skin? Unfortunately not.

Every time you use a dab of liquid soap to clean your hands, rub shampoo into your scalp, or spray perfume on your neck, your skin is absorbing that body care product like a sponge soaking up water on a kitchen countertop. Scientists believe that the skin absorbs up to 60 percent of everything applied to it and sends those substances directly into the bloodstream. This is the reason why more and more pharmaceuticals—such as hormone replacement therapy or nicotine suppression medications—are being delivered in a transdermal system through patches and creams.

Because of the body's ability to absorb compounds so well through the skin, I believe the cosmetic and personal care products we use are an often overlooked yet critical aspect of our overall health. How critical? Believe it or not, I think you have to be even more careful about what you put *on* your skin than what you put *into* your body.

People don't think too much about the body's epidermis, but they should. The skin is the largest organ of your body as well as an eliminative channel responsible for one-fourth of the body's daily detoxification. Often called the "third kidney" because of its cleansing role, the skin covers approximately two square yards of surface area and has the unique ability to *take in* beneficial compounds as well as to *release* toxins.

For instance, the skin synthesizes vitamin D from the ultraviolet rays of sunlight, which plays a vital role in immunity and blood cell formation, and releases contaminants through perspiration, be it from exercise and physical exertion to working outside under a hot sun or sitting inside an infrared sauna. I believe in the detoxification benefits of perspiration, which is why I often start my day with intense bursts of exercise followed by a session in my home sauna.

Since the Maker's Diet Revolution is all about building and cleansing, caring for your skin can uniquely unlock your health potential. Sure, the body has other ways to eliminate waste products when it's trying to cleanse. The lungs obtain oxygen from the air and remove carbon dioxide and other wastes from the bloodstream. The kidneys, liver, and lymphatic system certainly filter out toxins and target them for removal through the digestive tract via the large intestine.

The best approach, however, is to never introduce these toxins into your body in the first place. A great place to start on this path would be addressing what you put on your hair, skin, and nails.

If you haven't taken the time to learn about the toxins lurking in skin and body care products previously, now would be a good time to start.

THE SEARCH INTENSIFIES

My beautiful wife, Nicki, wants to look her best, just like millions of other American women. She's always been aboard my health train, except in one area that proved to be problematic—the use of conventional skin and body care products.

After we married, Nicki switched over to a predominantly organic, toxic-free diet. Finding non-toxic facial cleansers, toners, body lotions, moisturizers, shampoo, hairspray, and makeup, however, was a different story. She couldn't find any natural mascara, lipstick, or lip liner that she liked. The hairspray from the health food store left her hair feeling sticky, and she never liked the crunchy hair look.

In the book we wrote together in 2006, *The Great Physician's Prescription for Women's Health*, Nicki said this:

> I haven't been able to find organic makeup or hairspray that I like, but I will continue searching because I know I should be avoiding the toxins that these products contain. Even though

it's been a challenge to find organic substitutes for everyday cosmetics and toiletries, I expect organic skin care options to improve as the market for them grows bigger. I'm hoping that Jordan and his research team will develop more effective and usable products. I agree with my husband that it's a worthwhile goal to minimize your exposure to potentially harmful toxins whenever you can.

Nicki is like any woman who wants to look her best, but when it came to non-toxic skin care, body care, hair care, and makeup, she couldn't find organic, toxic-free substitutes that she liked. Nothing seemed to strike a chord with her, even though I brought home dozens of samples from trade shows and health and wellness expos.

Meanwhile, she kept using her "regular" cosmetics, waiting to find something that smelled good and worked effectively. The problem with toxins is that they don't often present health challenges for years or even decades, so it's easy to turn a blind eye in the moment. Nicki wasn't willing to use an organic skin and body care product unless it actually worked.

I'm sure this will come as no great revelation to you, but men and women are different when it comes to lotions, gels, shampoos, and conditioners. When they say the average American uses twelve different cosmetic products daily, I think the average balances out to women beating the guys by the score of 21-3! For years, I used *one* personal care product to wash my hands, soap up in the shower, and wash my hair. I even brushed my teeth with this one product when I ran out of my organic toothpaste. Like 99 percent of the male populace, I just wasn't a cosmetics guy.

But I knew skin and body care products were important to Nicki as well as nearly every female above the age of twelve. When Nicki and I took our trip to South Africa, I remember seeing a line of organic skin care products at a small farmer's market. I read the ingredient labels and liked what I saw, and since I was having no luck finding or developing a safe and effective line of skin and body care products in the States, I bought two extra suitcases and filled them with this South African skin care line. Unfortunately, even though the ingredients were stellar, the small group of women who tried the products found them less than desirable.

Some six years later, I decided it was time once again to attempt to develop a solution to the need for toxic-free skin and body care. After seeing research showing the average person, particularly female, uses fifteen to twenty-five personal care products daily, I knew we had to act. If you're touching between fifteen to twenty-five personal care products plus a dizzying number of cleaning products daily—dish soap, dishwasher detergent, laundry washing powder, bleach, floor cleaner, floor polish, floor wax remover, and floor wipes, etc.—then you're probably exposing yourself to 200 different chemicals.

Everything you touch or get on your skin is absorbed through your pores and goes right into your bloodstream. That's a noteworthy difference from how toxins—I'm thinking of pesticides on fruit, fungal toxins on grains, or preservatives and artificial colors in processed foods—enter your mouth through the food you eat and beverages you drink. Orally consumed toxins go through the body's filtering systems—the kidneys and liver—and are processed into less toxic substances before being sent to the bladder or bowels for elimination.

When you touch a household product or rub a lotion onto your skin, however, the toxins enter the body's bloodstream first—and rather quickly at that. I recently found a study showing that 49 percent of the carcinogenic pesticide DDT, which is found in cosmetics that contain lanolin, is absorbed via the skin and therefore into the bloodstream. Once those toxins start moving around the body, they can accumulate in places such as your fatty tissues and lymph nodes, including breast tissue.

I'm telling you, it's not good news out there with all these toxins in our personal care and cleaning products. A recent survey by the National Institute of Occupational Safety and Health analyzed 2,983 chemicals in personal care and cleaning products and determined that:

- over 800 were toxic

- nearly 800 caused acute toxicity, which means a rapid reaction

- 314 caused a biological mutation in the living system of the body

- 376 caused skin and eye irritation

- 148 could cause tumors in laboratory animals

- 218 caused reproductive complications

The nearly 3,000 chemicals that were analyzed were just the tip of the proverbial iceberg. It's estimated that 10,000 chemicals are routinely used in cosmetic products alone, but only 11 percent have been assessed for their health and safety by the FDA or other government agencies. The Environmental Working Group's Skin Deep Database states that one-third of all personal care products contain at least one chemical that has been linked to cancer.

Because the personal care industry is under-regulated—in contrast with the pharmaceutical and nutritional supplement industries, which are heavily regulated by governmental agencies such as the Food and Drug Administration—many people are unaware of the toxic chemicals in their everyday cosmetics and toiletries. You either have to be a biochemistry major or one determined consumer to decipher the incomprehensible list of multisyllabic ingredients labeled on the side of the container. Manufacturers use the longest words possible to throw you off the scent. Nowhere on the label will you find an explanation of how these ingredients work, leaving health-conscious folks in the dark.

Let me shine some light on the situation. I've already mentioned how phthalates are chemicals commonly used to preserve cosmetics and fragrances. Emerging scientific evidence is raising serious concerns about phthalates, showing a wide range of adverse effects in laboratory animals, including birth defects. U.S. testing indicates that phthalates are retained in human tissue at much higher levels than previously thought.

Chemicals commonly used in makeup, moisturizers, shampoos, shaving gels, and other cosmetics are parabens, which can increase the risk of breast cancer and male reproductive problems. Sodium lauryl sulfate, or SLS, is a surfactant (which reduces surface tension in the product) that is used extensively in shampoos, soaps, and toothpastes. SLS can irritate the skin for up to a week, causing free radicals and inflammation, while damaging skin proteins and healthy skin oils. Triclosan is used in many antibacterial soaps and other personal care items, such as deodorants and mouthwashes. This chemical has been linked to muscle function impairments in humans. Triclosan reduces contractions in cardiac and skeletal muscles, which can potentially contribute to heart disease and heart failure.

I could go on and on—just like those super-long ingredient lists on the back of shampoo bottles. Bottom line, these toxins shouldn't enter our bodies, or those of our children. When I think what's in baby shampoos—the ones that advertise "no tears"—it makes me want to cry. These baby shampoos contain anesthetizing ingredients as well as artificial dyes and parabens, which act as chemical preservatives. Laboratory tests commissioned by the Campaign for Safe Cosmetics and the Environmental Working Group showed that a mind-boggling 61 percent of children's bath products, including shampoos, contained both 1,4-dioxane and formaldehyde—two highly dangerous toxins linked to cancer, skin allergies, and more. Talk about toxins for tots.

As the parent of three young children and the husband of a wife I love, I knew we had to step up our efforts to create a line of skin and body care products. After much trial and effort, I believed we succeeded. I knew there were millions of other families just like us seeking the tools to reduce their exposure to dangerous chemicals.

I'll introduce our Beyond Organic Advanced Anti-Aging and Beyond Body Care products momentarily, but let me make a personal observation first. I'm getting older, in my late thirties, and I'm in a field where people do judge a book by its cover. What I'm trying to say is I have to look the part—walk the walk, if you will. I don't want to be one of those people who stands before a camera twenty-five years from now and says, "I'm sixty-three years old, but I'm all natural."

In other words, I don't want to have a facelift or laser peel. I want my skin to be clear, unblotched, and firm as I age—without potentially dangerous plastic surgery.

Now that we've released our Beyond Organic Anti-Aging and Beyond Body Care products, I've been all over them like brown on rice (a health food enthusiast's joke). You show me a process that leads to results, even one that takes six or seven steps, and I'll follow it. And with my new daily skin care regimen, I've been very diligent.

One time recently, Nicki walked into our master bathroom while I was doing my evening anti-aging skin care routine.

"Jordan, I've got to tell you something," she said.

"Honey, give me two or three minutes. I'm exfoliating."

You wouldn't have heard me say that a year ago. I don't think I even knew what "exfoliating" meant.

That all changed for me, and I hope it changes for you.

THE BEYOND ORGANIC SKIN AND BODY CARE PRODUCTS

When Beyond Organic began the process of creating a skin and body care system, we realized that the first benchmark was making products that were free of toxins. We sought and received the prestigious Certified ToxicFree designation from the ToxicFree Foundation, a private, nonprofit organization dedicated to educating the public about toxic ingredients in personal care, cosmetics, and household cleaning products. Then, ToxicFree Foundation evaluates chemicals and compounds used in skin and body care products for their toxicity, both long term and acute.

We also made sure that we utilized certified organic ingredients as much as possible, including our botanical extracts and essential oils. If an ingredient was not organic, we sought out one that was wildcrafted or carried the Ecocert designation. Ecocert is an international organization that independently tests ingredients to determine their impact on the environment and the body, as well as the presence of certified organic ingredients.

The Beyond Organic skin and body care product lines consist of certified organic, wildcrafted, Ecocert, and natural ingredients to give you efficacy as well as safety. This is something very rare in the skin and body care world, but we believe we have achieved exactly what we set out to do.

Flowing through the Beyond Organic skin and body care system is Reign Supreme, our structured spring water. Reign Supreme is our pristine spring water coming out of the mountains of north Georgia. It's one of the purest waters on record, having an extremely low level of total dissolved solids (TDS). Structured spring water provides an ideal delivery vehicle for nutrients and compounds to the cellular level.

The water that you consume, as well as apply to your skin when used in the making of lotions, creams, and cosmetics, is critical. Reign Supreme is naturally energized as well as structured, allowing the water molecules to penetrate and drive the nutrients and healthy compounds contained in Beyond Organic's skin and body care products into layers of your skin where they're needed.

The Beyond Organic skin and body care system is broken up into two product lines. We have our Anti-Aging skin care line and our Beyond Body Care system. Our Anti-Aging skin care line is an eight-piece system designed to help you look healthier and feel healthier. You'll have that glow, as they say, while providing critical nutrients, antioxidants, and other compounds directly to your skin, using a proprietary delivery system and cutting-edge ingredients.

Let's start with the **Beyond Organic Anti-Aging Botanical Cleanser**, which is a mild facial cleaner with antioxidants and nutrients to soothe and to cleanse deeply. Remember how I said that my idea of a skin-care regimen was to use the same product to wash my hands, my face, and use as a body wash and shampoo/conditioner in the shower?

Now that I've passed my mid-thirties, I knew it was time to put those old ways behind me and get serious about cleansing my skin. The Anti-Aging Botanical Cleanser is just the ticket for me and should be for you, too. Designed to be used twice daily, our Botanical Cleanser is safe for the eyes and can also be used as a detoxifying scalp treatment following shampoo and conditioner.

We use an organic and wildcrafted infusion that contains white tea leaf extract and extracts of biblical fruits such as dates, figs, olives, and pomegranates. Another ingredient in the infusion is wildcrafted hickory bark and sediments, or silt, from fresh water glaciers.

You might be wondering, *What in the world is glacial silt?*

I'm glad you asked. Underneath mountaintop glaciers, there's a dark, mud-like substance that's rich in color and has a silky feeling. Believe me, glacial silt is a unique ingredient with unique health properties. Everything in our Botanical Cleanser is delivered with Reign Supreme structured spring water. We use an organic essential oil blend that includes neroli (orange flower oil), organic lavender, an organic coconut oil with a vanilla infusion, organic tonka bean seed oil, and an organic immortelle oil, which is a powerful tonic mushroom.

Please note that our Anti-Aging Botanical Cleanser does not contain common chemical agents that are considered toxic. These would include propylene glycols, polyethylene glycols (also known as PEGs), sodium laurel sulfates (or SLS), triclosan (which is common in most anti-microbial cleansers), monoethanaolamine (also known as MEA), or artificial colors or fragrances.

Step 2 in the Beyond Organic Anti-Aging system is our **Beyond Organic Anti-Aging Neroli Toner**, which balances and calms all skin types from dry to oily. A major ingredient is neroli floral water, which promotes a healthy mood and positive outlook.

Spotlighting the ingredients in the Anti-Aging Neroli Toner, we have, once again, included our organic, wildcrafted botanical infusion with a biblical extract of date, fig, olive, and pomegranate, wildcrafted hickory bark, and fresh water glacial silt. All are delivered with Reign Supreme structured spring water.

We use organic aloe vera leaf juice, which has been used for skin health for thousands of years. Neroli orange floral water is a key ingredient, as well as an Ecocert green clay extract from France. Clay, just like the glacial silt, is known for the way it absorbs unhealthy compounds. I've been a fan of clay, used topically and taken orally, for years. French green clay is one of the most extraordinary compounds on the planet because of its unique ability to pull toxins into itself for easy removal from the body.

We also use a botanical preservation system with two types of Japanese honeysuckle flower extracts. Instead of adding chemical toxic preservatives, we found a preservation system that actually benefits the body. Neroli Toner is best used immediately after cleansing, twice daily prior to moisturizing.

Step 3 in our Anti-Aging system is our **Beyond Organic Anti-Aging Radiant Serum**, which is used twice daily for deep repairing and firming action. When using, allow thirty to sixty seconds to penetrate before following with one of our two moisturizers, AM Moisturizer for the morning or Replenishing Night Cream for the evening.

With the Anti-Aging Radiant Serum, you'll find certified toxic-free ingredients from organic wildcrafted and Ecocert sources. This is one product that makes an immediate difference on your skin that you can feel. Some of the ingredients in the Anti-Aging Radiant Serum include an organic, wildcrafted botanical infusion with aloe leaf extract, the four biblical fruits, wildcrafted hickory bark, and fresh water glacial silt along with Reign Supreme structured spring water.

In our Anti-Aging Radiant Serum, we have a unique clinically studied ingredient called a biomimetic peptide blend. This peptide, or protein, is designed to mimic the protein found in your skin that can restore your skin to great health. This biomimetic peptide blend boosts collagen production, and collagen is an important protein found in your skin and other parts of your body, providing a significant reduction in the appearance of fine lines and wrinkles.

This peptide blend assists in creating optimal skin structural support and activates natural skin rejuvenation. We add powerful ingredients such as broccoli seed oil, an organic essential oil blend, and sea buckthorn oil, all of which help provide the skin and other parts of the body with powerful fatty acids.

Once again, our Anti-Aging Radiant Serum does not contain toxic chemical ingredients.

Step 4 in the skin care regimen is using our **Beyond Organic Anti-Aging AM Moisturizer**. In the morning, after cleansing, toning, and applying your Radiant Serum, gently massage this AM Moisturizer on your face, neck, and hands. One of the key ingredients is argan oil, which is highly prized for its anti-aging properties and possesses a remarkable ability to nourish, moisturize, and improve skin elasticity. Argan oil effectively reduces the appearance of wrinkles and fine lines and regulates the skin's natural oils at a healthy level.

Key ingredients in AM Moisturizer include the organic, wildcrafted botanical infusion with white tea leaf extract, date, fig, olive, and pomegranate, wildcrafted hickory bark, glacial silt, Reign Supreme structured spring water, and broccoli seed oil, which helps prevent skin damage from UV radiation. Broccoli seeds are rich in sulforaphane, which is a sulfur-based compound wonderful for the body.

Step 5 in the anti-aging system includes **Beyond Organic Replenishing Night Cream**, which is used in the evenings the same way you use AM Moisturizer in the morning. That bit of information is for all you guys out there who are novices like myself.

In the evening, after cleansing, toning, and applying your Radiant Serum, apply this nourishing moisturizer for deep repair and rejuvenation. The Replenishing Night Cream stimulates the skin's defense mechanisms against oxidative stress that you've experienced during the day.

The Replenishing Night Cream is a rich cream that helps remove toxins and oxidative stress that cause advanced symptoms of aging. Key ingredients include organic aloe vera leaf juice, organic wildcrafted botanical infusion, and organic beech tree bud extract, which has been shown to improve oxygen consumption by 71 percent.

Oxygen is wonderful—we can't live without it—but oxygen is a free radical when it's in a certain form and in a certain amount. Antioxidants consume oxygen, which is a form of oxidation. When organic beech tree bud extract improves oxygen consumption, you'll see a boost in skin moisturization.

The addition of argan kernel oil helps to nourish, moisturize, and improve skin elasticity and reduce the appearance of wrinkles and fine lines. We also added organic shea butter to promote skin health. As with all of our Beyond Organic anti-aging products, Replenishing Night Cream does not contain toxic chemical ingredients.

Step 6 in our anti-aging system is our **Beyond Organic Anti-Aging Eye Cream**, which you can apply twice daily under and around the eyes. I must admit that this was a new experience for me, but I really enjoy using it. Best used after the AM or PM Moisturizer, this skin care product will make a big difference in the health of skin for men and women.

The Anti-Aging Eye Cream supports the reduction of wrinkles, dark circles, and under-eye puffiness. You'll notice that this cream is rich but not too heavy for the delicate skin around the eyes. You don't need a lot, but it's very well absorbed.

Our Anti-Aging Eye Cream is toxic-free, using powerful organic safflower oleosomes, ingredients that help penetrate and, in a sense, organize the key lipids within your skin cells. Safflower oleosomes have been shown to improve skin health by building the skin barrier faster.

People say all the time that when you have dry skin, you should hydrate—drink a lot of water. But have you ever seen a damaged wood deck? That damage came from water, most likely, so the best way to restore your wood deck is not by washing it down with more water but by using oil.

Here's how a damaged wood deck relates to skin care. I believe, as do many, that the most important element to determine how young and vibrant that you look depends on how you maintain the proper lipids or oils contained in and on your skin. One ingredient that helps maintain and retain skin lipids is safflower oleosomes.

We also use an Amazon jungle trio—Brazilian ginseng, Madonna Lily, and Muira Puama—that is Ecocert certified. The overall reduction of cellulite appearance by using this jungle trio was 57 percent from a volunteer panel after thirty days. That's right—57 percent of people using this ingredient said they had an overall reduction of cellulite, often found on your thighs but can also be found under your eyes. This product really works.

For Step 7, perhaps one of the most exciting formulations is our **Beyond Organic Anti-Aging Lift Serum**. The people in our test and focus groups probably had more to say about the Anti-Aging Lift Serum than any formulation we have. Here's a product that provides advanced support in the Beyond Organic anti-aging system. Key ingredients in the Anti-Aging Lift Serum have been shown to prevent deep wrinkles and even to repair existing damage by strengthening the skin's connective tissue. Formulated for intense firming action and concentrated anti-aging power, the Anti-Aging Lift Serum will be a favorite for everyone who wants an immediate feeling of healthier, tighter skin.

Our Anti-Aging Lift Serum contains an organic, wildcrafted, botanical infusion and a sea vegetable blend that has been shown to inhibit free radicals that cause cellular damage—by up to 22 percent. The nice blue-green color comes from the mineral element malachite, which has been shown to increase the amount of collagen and elastin, two key proteins in your skin that are produced by the fibroblast cells.

We also have a biomimetic peptide blend, which, in clinical studies, showed an improvement in the skin's elasticity in 93 percent of participants with 92 percent of users noting firmer, fuller, and denser skin. We also have a blend of bamboo, green tea, and glucosamine that showed 45 percent improvement in reducing fine lines and wrinkles. The glucosamine is enzyme-produced, not from shellfish. Once again, our Anti-Aging Lift Serum does not contain toxic chemical ingredients.

Continuing on to Step 8, the **Beyond Organic Anti-Aging Açai Exfoliator** rounds out our advanced anti-aging system. Designed to support your skin in many ways, the fruit acids, plants, and mineral exfoliators and açai pulp work together for gentle yet thorough exfoliation.

Numerous botanical agents in Açai Exfoliator soothe the skin while providing antioxidant benefits during your skin exfoliation, which should happen two or three times a week. The Anti-Aging Açai Exfoliator contains organic aloe vera leaf juice, the organic wildcrafted botanical infusion that is key to many of our formulas. Organic açai pulp and pumice flower, which is a mineral that provides mild but effective exfoliating action, are also part of the formulation.

Many exfoliating products use beads that are plastic or made from petrochemicals, where our formula uses only naturally derived ingredients. We also use a copper-rich chlorophyll called chlorophyllin, which is fantastic for your skin, plus organic wild hyssop and organic lemon and lime. These fruits and botanical acids are effective in removing dead skin cells.

THE BEYOND ORGANIC BODY CARE LINE

The Beyond Organic Body Care line is great for the entire family and provides variety in your own skin and body care regimen.

The first product is the **Beyond Body Care Hand and Body Lotion**, a luxurious lotion that revitalizes, rejuvenates, and hydrates your skin, protecting you from dryness, sun exposure, and stress. Only the very best toxic-free compounds are used to nourish your hands and your body. Our Beyond Body Care Hand and Body Lotion contains our organic, wildcrafted botanical infusion, but this time with some different ingredients.

These would be organic green tea leaf extract, jasmine, and Bulgarian rose, which is combined with wildcrafted hickory bark, Reign Supreme structured spring water, and two biblical essential oils—frankincense and myrrh. The addition of organic sea buckthorn oil and safflower oleosomes, macadamia nut oil, an essential oil blend containing oils of blood orange, bergamot, rose hip, and vanilla-infused coconut oil help keep the lipid barrier intact.

Our Beyond Body Care Hand and Body Lotion does not contain common chemical agents such as propylene glycol, polyethylene glycols, sodium lauryl sulfates (SLS), triclosan, artificial colors, or fragrances. This is a product you're going to want to apply after washing your hands or stepping out of the shower.

When you do need to wash your hands, reach for our **Beyond Organic Botanical Hand Wash,** which allows your hands to stay hydrated and preserve the delicate lipids and moisture. Our Beyond Body Care Botanical Hand Wash is free of harsh chemical detergents that strip the oils from the skin, right along with the dirt. We believe that you need to wash with a cleanser that will leave your hands feeling softer and better after washing.

You'll find certified, toxic-free ingredients in this tremendous formula. Our Botanical Hand Wash contains the organic, wildcrafted botanical infusion, providing green tea, jasmine, Bulgarian rose, wildcrafted hickory bark, Reign Supreme structured spring water, organic frankincense, and organic myrrh. That's not all: there's aloe vera leaf juice, organic

Canadian willow herb extract, and a blend of Ecocert açaí, passion fruit, and babassu seed oils, which comes from the babassu palm tree that grows in the Amazon region.

Please note that we've gone to all reaches of the planet to find these amazing, unique ingredients that are in every formula of our Beyond Organic skin and body care line. We use a slightly different essential oil blend that contains sweet orange, blood orange, bergamot, vanilla-infused coconut oil, pink grapefruit oil, and ginger oil. Once again, no common chemical agents that are considered toxic are present in any of our Beyond Organic skin and body care products.

Our **Beyond Body Care Sweet Orange Shampoo** is awesome and goes beyond ordinary shampoo by helping to unblock clogged follicles, moisturize the hair, and provide anti-microbial support. This shampoo can also be used as a soothing, toning, leave-in scalp treatment. The formula is made up of certified toxic-free ingredients that are organic wildcrafted and Ecocert certified.

Beyond Body Care Sweet Orange Shampoo contains an organic, wildcrafted botanical infusion, an organic essential oil blend, and Ecocert rice-based amino acids, which are the building blocks of protein because your hair is made largely of protein. Once again, no chemical toxic agents.

Folks, I challenge you to look at shampoos put out there by the big manufacturers. You will be shocked at what you're putting on your hair and your children's hair. Remember, even though the scalp is covered with hair in most instances, it's an ideal delivery vehicle for whatever is in your shampoo. The skin on your scalp is so absorbant that years ago I thought about coming up with a children's multivitamin delivered in the form of a shampoo.

Shampoo is always followed by conditioner, right? **Beyond Body Care Sweet Orange Conditioner** provides effective conditioning treatment, using organic oils and botanicals to help restore optimal moisture balance, smooth frayed hair cuticles, and help repair split ends. Beyond Body Care Sweet Orange Conditioner contains organic, wildcrafted botanical infusions, an organic essential oil blend, sweet almond oil, aloe vera leaf juice, açaí, passion fruit, babassu seed oils, and no toxic agents.

Our **Beyond Body Care Clean Citrus Shower Gel** is one of my favorite products because of the way this gentle botanical body cleanser washes away pollutants while the skin is soothed, moisturized, and protected against free radical damage.

Chlorine and other contaminants are often present in our municipal water supplies, which is why I recommend having a shower filter to remove chlorine, chloramines, and other toxins. Whether you do or don't have a shower filter, Clean Citrus Shower Gel will help you wash off any junk contained in the water, and your skin will feel fresh and healthy with this nutrient-rich, toxic-free shower gel. You can apply to wet skin in the shower or add to running water for a cleansing, soothing bath.

Beyond Body Care Clean Citrus Shower Gel contains organic, wild-crafted botanical infusions, an organic essential oil blend, and does not contain common chemicals.

Not too many people think of their lips when it comes to body care, and that included me. In years past, the only time I applied a lip balm was during a once-a-year ski trip to the Colorado Rockies. Since then, I've come to realize that it's important to keep your lips healthy and your lipid barrier intact. Why? Because when our lips dry out—such as when we're at high altitude—the normal response is to lick our lips as if the water in our saliva can add moisture. (It can't.)

The **Beyond Body Care Lip Balms** can help you restore the nutrients and components to provide healthy lips from chapping and being overly dry. Our lip balms come in two styles—**Triple Mint** and **Pomegranate Berry**—and contain certified non-toxic and certified organic ingredients. Our Triple Mint and Pomegranate Berry lip balms are wonderful for multiple, everyday use.

CLOSING THOUGHT

As I mentioned earlier, your skin is your largest organ. It's an eliminative organ, but it's also your body's first line of defense against the outside world. The health of your skin protects and even reflects the health of your body.

So when thinking about skin and body care, put your trust in products that help you feel and look your best without the toxic load that you and your family would rather avoid.

You'll be pleased with the results—both now and in years to come.

17

FUNCTIONAL FITNESS

Daniel seemed like a pretty tough guy, defying the government and even staring down lions. I wonder if he ever worked out with dumbbells or barbells, or better yet, swung kettlebells to stay in great shape.

I'm being facetious, of course, but I would imagine that Daniel and his colleagues Hananiah, Misha-el, and Azariah were supremely fit and in top physical shape. I say that for several reasons:

1. After King Nebuchadnezzar conquered Jerusalem, he ordered his right-hand man Ashpenaz to sift through Judah's noble families and "select only strong, healthy, and good-looking men" (Daniel 1:4 NLT). Other translations called them "young men without any physical defect" (NIV) or "no blemish" (NKJV).

2. Once singled out, Daniel and his friends didn't board a bus, take a train, or enjoy a leisurely plane flight from Jerusalem to Babylon. They walked. How far? The remains of Babylon, the city-state of ancient Mesopotamia, are found in present-day Al Hillah in the Babil Province of Iraq, about fifty-two miles south of Baghdad. My research shows that the distance from Jerusalem to Babylon is 543 miles across a dusty desert.

3. Once they arrived in Babylon, there's no mention in the Book of Daniel of the four pumping iron or going out on an early morning jog, but I would imagine that they didn't sit around

King Nebuchadnezzar's palace with their noses buried in papyrus all day. They were kept on the go.

Imagine the difference between Daniel and those living in Babylon, circa 605 B.C., and Americans today, where our eating habits and sedentary lifestyles have produced a populace that's soft around the middle, among other places. Most people can't even be bothered to park and walk a hundred feet into their favorite fast food restaurant; instead, they stay in their cars and breeze by the drive-thru lane.

While the main focus of the Maker's Diet Revolution is nutrition, physical fitness is also essential to good health. In fact, the right kind of exercise is one of the best things you can do for your body, mind, and spirit. Exercise can be both a cleansing *and* building activity: pumping those legs and arms speeds up the heart and makes you breathe faster, which helps transfer oxygen from your lungs to your bloodstream and increases the body's natural immune system function. Exercise stimulates the important white blood cells in your body to move from the organs into the bloodstream, where they can mount a defense against invaders and toxins inside the body. Exercise also builds strength and endurance, two attributes in dwindling supply nowadays.

Judging from statistics, consistent exercise is an extremely difficult challenge for most people these days.

I've always enjoyed exercising. In my early twenties, I was a certified fitness instructor, and nearly seventeen years later I still love to exercise. But like any father with three children under the age of ten and a lot going on outside the home, there are times when I need to be more...efficient with my routine.

Some mornings, I do an intense workout using combination sets that takes as little as twelve minutes. The combination of high reps, moderate weights, and high-intensity super sets helps me build muscle and lose fat while increasing oxygen uptake. I also love the fact that I'm burning fat for hours after the workout because I exercise on an empty stomach, which causes my body to use stored fat for energy. That's a double bonus. Remember, I don't eat my first meal until after noon at the earliest, so I'm still cleansing in the morning.

If you're like me and don't have a lot of free time to work out, then this type of exercise—known as functional interval training, surge training, or burst training—could be just the ticket. Burst training involves exercising at 90 percent to 100 percent of your maximum effort for thirty to sixty seconds in order to burn your body's stored sugar, which is known as glycogen, followed by thirty to sixty seconds of low impact for recovery. Burst training is long on exertion and short on duration.

A good friend of mine, Dr. Josh Axe, author, radio host, and chiropractic physician, has developed a great program utilizing the principles of burst training. Dr. Axe has served as a wellness physician to many professional athletes and celebrities and has a passion for delivering maximum results in limited time.

I asked Dr. Axe to explain burst training and his brand new fitness program he calls BurstFIT. Here is what he had to say:

> I think burst training is a great way to experience fast fat loss.
>
> Most people who want to burn fat and lose weight assume that going to the gym and doing traditional aerobic exercise such as pacing yourself on an elliptical machine or jogging on a treadmill is the best way to see results. But recent research is proving that long distance cardiovascular exercise is *not* the fastest way to burn fat and lose weight.
>
> If you've been spending hours on the treadmill and not seeing any results, it's because long-distance cardiovascular exercise can decrease testosterone and raise the levels of stress hormones such as cortisol. Increased levels of cortisol stimulate the appetite, increase fat storage, and slow down or even inhibit exercise recovery.
>
> A recent study in *Psychoneuroendocrinology* showed evidence of long-term high cortisol levels in aerobic endurance athletes. Researchers tested levels of cortisol in 304 endurance athletes (runners, cyclists, and triathletes) and compared them to non-athletes. The results showed higher cortisol levels with higher training. *The*

Journal of Sports Sciences found that long periods of aerobic exercise increased oxidative stress leading to chronic inflammation.

If you want to see results fast without the negative effects of traditional cardiovascular exercise, your best option is burst training. Burst training, also known as interval training, combines short, high intensity bursts of exercise with slow recovery phases, repeated during one exercise session. Burst training is done at 85 to 100 percent maximum heart rate rather than 50 to 70 percent in moderate endurance activity.

With burst and other types of interval training, you are getting the same cardiovascular benefits as endurance exercise but without the negative side effects in much shorter time period. Essentially, burst training is exercising like a sprinter rather than a marathon runner.

One of the major benefits of burst training is that it can be done in the comfort of your own home with zero or minimal equipment. An example of burst training would be going to a track and walking the curves and sprinting the straightaways. Or getting on a spin bike and cycling hard for 20 seconds then going easy for 20 seconds then repeating that effort for between five to forty minutes.

Burst training isn't necessarily new. Elite athletes and Olympians have known this secret to exercising and have been practicing interval training for years. The research proves that anybody—not just elite athletes—can utilize interval training and achieve amazing results.

Research from the University of New South Wales Medical Sciences found that burst cardio could burn up to three times more body fat than moderate cardio. The researchers studied two groups and found that the group who did eight seconds of sprinting on a bike, followed by twelve seconds of exercising lightly for twenty minutes, lost *three times* as much fat as other women, who exercised at a continuous, regular pace for forty minutes.

The reason burst training works is because it produces a unique metabolic response in your body. Intermittent sprinting causes your body not to burn high amounts of fat during exercise, but after exercise, your metabolism stays elevated and will continue to burn fat for the next twenty-four to forty-eight hours!

In addition, chemicals called catecholamines are produced that allow even more fat to be burned. This causes increased fat oxidation, which drives greater weight loss. By the way, the women in the study lost the most weight off their legs and buttocks.

Another study published in the *Journal of Applied Physiology* in April 2007 researched eight different women in their early twenties. They were told to cycle for ten sets of four minutes of hard riding, followed by two minutes of rest.

After two weeks, the amount of fat burned increased by 36 percent, and their cardiovascular fitness improved by 13 percent.

The key benefits of burst training can be summed up in this manner:

- Burst training can burn up to three times more body fat than traditional or moderate cardio.
- After two weeks of burst training, fat burning increases by 36 percent.
- Your body will continue to burn fat for the next twenty-four to forty-eight hours after you're done exercising.
- You can work out in less time and see better results.

Burst training…it's worth checking out.

IGNITE THAT FAT-BURNING FURNACE

Burst training is a type of functional interval training that I've recommended in my previous books, including *Perfect Weight America*. Not only do I see the value of shorter but more intense workout periods, but I've personally experienced the benefits of strengthening my heart and lungs, building muscle, and igniting my body's fat-burning furnace. I urge you to run—not walk—to your computer and check out burst training and start scorching both peripheral fat (found in arms, legs, and buttocks) and visceral fat (found in your torso, mainly the abdominal region) during and after your workout.

By sharply increasing and decreasing your heart rate, you'll burn more calories in a twenty-four-hour period than if you spend the same amount of time striding at the same pace on a treadmill. Burst training will improve your resting metabolic rate (RMR) as well as your VO_2 Max rate, which is the maximum amount of oxygen that can be used by an individual, in milliliters, in one minute per kilogram of body weight.

You see, you can't lose weight—or sustain the weight you've lost after completing the Daniel Diet—without stoking the body's furnace to burn up reserves of fat. When you complete a series of burst-type exercises, you increase your oxygen intake as well as your heart and lung capacity so that your body turns into a fat-burning engine that incinerates excess fat long after you've stopped working out.

You do this by building muscle—or restoring muscle that's been lost over the years—through functional, body-strengthening exercises. Even if you add a pound or two from gaining muscle, you'll be better off because one pound of muscle burns thirty to fifty calories a day while one pound of fat burns only three calories a day.

When the body exercises, it works in two basic ways: aerobically and anaerobically. The body is said to be working aerobically when it operates at a pace that allows the cardio-respiratory system—the lungs, heart, and bloodstream—to replenish energy as you exercise. Put another way, aerobic exercise causes the body to utilize oxygen to create energy. This is basically anything that gets the heart going, such as running on a treadmill, cycling on stationary bikes, or stepping on stair stepper machines.

Aerobic exercise is generally associated with non-resistance activities such as:

- aerobics classes
- basketball
- bicycling
- calisthenics

- dancing
- gardening
- golfing
- hiking on level terrain
- ice skating
- inline skating
- racquetball
- scuba diving
- snowboarding
- snow skiing
- soccer
- softball
- squash
- table tennis
- tennis
- volleyball
- walking
- water skiing.

Anaerobic exercise is any form of non-sustained physical activity that typically involves a limited number of specific muscles over a short period of time. Examples of anaerobic exercise are:

- lifting weights
- using strength-training machines such as Nautilus and Hoist
- jumping rope or jumping on a rebounder (depending on duration, can be aerobic as well)
- sprinting
- working the body's core muscles through the use of functional exercises with rubber bands, stability balls, medicine balls, and Russian kettlebells

I can explain the differences between aerobic and anaerobic exercise further by using a word picture. Let's say you've been exercising on a stationary bike all winter long at your fitness club. Your usual routine is to pedal two or three times a week for thirty-minute stints. Spring is in the air, so you decide to take advantage of the warm sun by going on an outdoor bike ride. The temperature is just right on this Saturday morning—around 70 degrees. It feels good to pedal briskly in the fresh air on a level bike path. You are performing classic aerobic exercise.

In the distance, you spot a series of hills. You pedal over the first one with little exertion, but you can feel it in your legs on the second hill. The final climb, however, is a killer: to keep up your cadence and speed, you stand on your pedals and give that little extra oomph to clear the rise.

What you've just done on Hill Number 3 is switch over from aerobic to anaerobic exercise. You handled the first two hills aerobically, but to maintain speed on the final rise, you needed extra help. When you stood on the pedals and pumped those tired leg muscles, you crossed a threshold and began exercising the body *anaerobically.*

Chances are you couldn't sustain that type of energy exertion very long since only elite athletes can do *any* form of anaerobic exercise beyond a few moments. Yet anaerobic exercise is the best way to build muscle and simultaneously burn fat. Many studies have shown that anaerobic exercise burns more calories and thus more fat than aerobic exercise—up to *five* times more, according to this Colorado State University study.

Calories Burned in Sixty Minutes of Exercise

Exercise	During exercise	Two hours after exercise	Three to fifteen hours after exercise
Aerobic	210	25	0
Anaerobic	650	150	260

As you can see, we're talking about a huge difference in caloric expenditures. What happens is that aerobic exercise typically burns 25 percent muscle and 75 percent fat for body energy, but anaerobic exercise burns 100 percent body fat for body energy.

The dirty little secret in the weight-loss world is that the first thing you lose when you diet—and casually exercise—is muscle tissue. Your body cannibalizes muscle tissue to support your energy needs, but the fat stays on your tummy and hips. Trying to lose weight without exercising anaerobically would be like running a 10K race with ankle weights: it's going to take you a lot longer to reach the finish line. It's extremely difficult to lose fat permanently without exercising anaerobically.

You can achieve your fitness goals as well as drop unwanted fat by incorporating burst training exercises into your lifestyle. But first I must issue a health advisory: burst training is not recommend for those new to exercise or out of shape. You may have to spend the first week or two, maybe your first month, getting your body reacquainted with physical exertion. You should walk on a treadmill, pedal a stationary bike, or jump on a rebounder before tackling intense, interval training.

So in this sense, it's a good idea to start slow and easy and make steady progress in your physical conditioning. Once you have a new or renewed foundation of fitness, then kick things up a notch by engaging in a burst training program.

Here are seven simple exercises that Dr. Axe recommends that you can do at home:

1. Run in place. Keep your knees high and the tempo fast. See if you can keep pumping your legs for an entire minute.

2. Jumping jacks. Sure, maybe the last you did jumping jacks was back in high school gym class, but you'll be reminded years later that simple jumping jacks weren't a waste of time. See how many jumping jacks you can do in thirty seconds.

3. Squat pulses. With your feet should-width apart, squat low and then straight up. Standing on a bosu ball while making squats will up the ante. Make sure your knees don't come past your toes.

4. Jump rope. Any grammar school kid can use a jump rope, right? If the last time you jumped rope was when you did jumping jacks, you might be surprised how difficult and efficient this simple exercise is.

5. Biking. You can bike in spin classes at your fitness club or outside on streets and roads, but spin classes are always going to be

better for burst training because the spin class leader will be after you to get those revolutions up.

6.   Swim. Like biking, you have to push yourself when you're in the pool.

7.   High jumps. Simply stand in place, reach your arms above your head, and jump as fast as you can for thirty to sixty seconds.

The key is giving it everything you've got—for a short time. And then resting. And doing it again and again until you're winded and need a longer rest. Twenty minutes or less is all you need to make burst training a substitute for the old paradigm of exercise.

Of course, if you belong to a fitness or athletic club, you can tap into various high intensity classes that fit the burst training approach. Zumba is a dance fitness craze that seems to be working for many exercise enthusiasts. Cardio muscle classes keep you moving while lifting dumbbells; step aerobic classes is a choreographed routine of stepping up and down a rectangular platform; and spin classes have you performing interval training on a stationary bike. You can seek out studios that specialize in Pilates, a body conditioning routine that can be very intense.

GOTTA HAVE MORE KETTLEBELL

My favorite tool for anaerobic exercise is the Russian kettlebell, which looks like an oversized cannonball with a handle. Kettlebells are an excellent way to work the body's "core" muscles. When you swing and lift kettlebells, you're the beneficiary of one of those old-school workouts that really get the heart pumping and stimulate the key muscles of the body.

I began training with kettlebells in 2007 when Pavel Tsatsouline, a Russian who trained Red Army Special Forces back in the day, gave me personal instruction on how to use this powerful tool. Pavel had immigrated to the United States in the 1990s determined to put kettlebells on the map, and I'd say he's succeeded. Ever since I received my first set of kettlebells six years ago, I've been using them almost exclusively in my morning workout programs.

Kettlebells are different from free weights because their handles give them a displaced center of gravity. They come in various weights from 10 to 106 pounds. What I like about kettlebells and Pavel's unique training sequences is their efficacy and efficiency. Kettlebell training involves exercises that engage the entire body, making traditional Olympic lifts such as snatches, clean and jerks, and dead lifts more functional.

Technique is very important when training with Russian kettlebells. A great beginning exercise is holding a kettlebell by the horns, chest-height, and performing knee bends called goblet squats, keeping your weight on your heels. One-arm kettlebell swinging "is the closest thing to throwing a punch," says Pavel, which must be a reason why kettlebells are a very popular training tool for boxers and mixed martial artists.

My nine-year-old son Joshua works out with kettlebells, and I'm amazed how quickly he's learned proper technique. Likewise, Nicki has become proficient in kettlebell exercises.

The kettlebells I use are the original bells brought to the U.S. by Pavel and distributed by Dragon Door. For more information on Russian kettlebell training, visit www.dragondoor.com.

MOVING ON

Performing bursts of intense exercises that push the body will help you make great gains in strength, balance, and flexibility. Exercise is essential for cleansing and building the body and is a vital component of the Maker's Diet Revolution. Without exercise, you won't achieve or maintain optimal physical health.

Exercise is essential to maintaining any weight loss you experience during the 10-Day Daniel Diet. When you exercise, you're helping the body remove toxins through breathing more deeply, which releases toxins from the lungs and from perspiration that releases toxins from your lymphatic system.

I think—and this is coming from a very busy guy—that the toughest thing about exercise is not the exertion it demands but finding time to do it consistently. You'll have to set your mind to getting the body moving again. You'll have to discipline yourself. The good news is that you don't have to spend a lot of hours exercising.

By utilizing burst training as recommended by Dr. Axe or incorporating Russian kettlebells into a high-intensity, short-duration training routine, you can build a healthy body in just minutes a day.

18

THE MAKER'S DIET REVOLUTION: YOUR DAILY PLAN

I hope, after reading the previous seventeen chapters, that you're inspired and motivated to take your health to the next level by joining the Maker's Diet Revolution.

In this chapter, you will find great information to help you on your journey. I've included a sample three-day eating plan that incorporates the daily cleansing principles as well as shopping tips to help you locate and purchase healthful foods and beverages for your family. You'll also receive dining out tips so you can enjoy socializing with friends without sacrificing your health.

THE MAKER'S DIET REVOLUTION PLAN

During each day on the Maker's Diet Revolution Plan, you'll be eating during a six- to eight-hour time frame. While the diet allows for great freedom in the amount of food consumed during the allotted time, I encourage you to consume foods in the following order: when going from your daily cleansing to building (eating) phase, I recommend that you start your meal by consuming a raw fresh food such as cultured veggies or a raw salad.

Next, consume an entrée containing a good portion of high-quality proteins and fats and high-fiber cooked veggies. If you choose to consume a starchy carbohydrate such as a whole grain or sweet potato, or something sweet such as a piece of fruit, that should come toward the end of your meal.

Disclaimers Regarding Raw Dairy, Raw Eggs, Raw Fish, and Raw Juice

The following are government-issued warnings for the consumption of raw or undercooked foods and beverages.

- Raw milk products may contain disease-causing microorganisms. Persons at highest risk for of disease from these organisms include newborns and infants, the elderly, pregnant women, those taking corticosteroids, antibiotics and antacids, and those having chronic illnesses and other conditions that weaken their immunity.

- Consuming raw or undercooked eggs may increase your risk of food-borne illness.

- Consuming raw or undercooked seafood may increase your risk of food-borne illness.

- Juice that has not been pasteurized may contain bacteria that can increase the risk of food-borne illness. People most at risk are children, the elderly, and persons with a weakened immune system.

Note: I am the founder of Beyond Organic and Garden of Life, and, where applicable, I am recommending these companies' products. Regarding other companies that I recommend, I do so because I consume their products and find them to be of good nutritional quality and taste. Beyond Organic and Garden of Life cannot be held responsible for the quality or claims of these products. Please do your research and consult with your healthcare practitioner prior to starting any new diet or supplement program.

Important Disclaimer

This chapter is not intended to provide medical advice or to take the place of medical advice and treatment from your personal physician. Readers are advised to consult their own doctors or other qualified health professionals regarding treatment of their medical problems.

Neither the publisher nor the author takes any responsibility for any possible consequences from any treatment, action, or application of medicine, supplement, herb, or preparation to any person reading or following the information in this book. If readers are taking prescription medications, they should consult with their physicians before beginning any nutrition or supplementation program.

The order in which you eat your meal is very important and can make a significant difference in your health.

Speaking of carbohydrates, they are the sugars and starches contained in plant foods, and while they can be an important part of a well-rounded diet, our modern-day eating regimen revolves around sweetened or sugared foods such as breakfast cereals, blueberry muffins, cookies, ice cream, and flavored coffees.

The predominant form of carbohydrate contained in grains, fluid dairy products, sugar, potatoes, and corn are known as disaccharides. A disaccharide is a "double sugar" that is composed of two single sugar (monosaccharide) molecules linked to each other. When you consume too much refined white sugar, white flour, and even "healthy" whole food forms of disaccharide-rich foods, you're feeding the "bad" microorganisms in your gut and upsetting the balance of the intestinal flora—prompting digestive problems to strike.

The MDR Daily Plan will likely have you cutting back on your starches considerably. I know that avoiding or limiting sugar and its sweet relatives—high fructose corn syrup, sucrose, molasses, and maple syrup—is easier said than done, but all those sweets can turn your health sour!

The carbohydrates you want to consume are low glycemic, high nutrient, low sugar, and high in monosaccharides. These would be mostly high-fiber fruits, especially berries, vegetables, nuts, seeds, and some legumes.

Eating unrefined carbohydrate-containing foods introduces important nutrients, antioxidants, and fiber into your body. Fiber is the indigestible remnants of plant cells found in vegetables, fruits, whole grains, nuts, seeds, and beans. Fiber-rich foods take longer to break down and are partially indigestible, which means that as these foods work their way through the digestive tract, they absorb water and increase the elimination of waste in the large intestine.

Good sources of fiber are:

- berries

- fruits with edible skins (apples, pears, and grapes)

- citrus fruits

- whole non-gluten grains (amaranth, millet, quinoa, and buckwheat), and soaked and/or sprouted whole grains are even more digestible

- green peas

- carrots

- cucumbers

- zucchini

- tomatoes

Green leafy vegetables such as spinach and micro greens are also fiber-rich.

You'll see in the approved foods lists that white sugar, artificial sweeteners, and preservatives are forbidden. If you're currently consuming high amounts of carbohydrates and/or artificial sweeteners on a regular basis, reducing the amounts may cause temporary withdrawal-type symptoms such as headaches, dry mouth, carbohydrate cravings, less energy, mood swings, or even changes in your bowel habits. These "detox" reactions are indications that the program is working as the body attempts to cleanse toxins from the system. When you have the "blahs," increase water intake and rest.

This plan restricts the amounts of disaccharide-heavy carbohydrate foods such as pastas and breads but makes up for it in the variety of delicious, filling foods you can enjoy.

The MDR Daily Plan will have you avoid unhealthy fats and proteins that have deleterious effects on the body. This includes the avoidance of dairy products containing a protein known as A1 beta-casein, which can cause dairy intolerance in many individuals. In addition, limit or avoid alcoholic beverages—wine, beer, or spirits.

When following the MDR Daily Plan, consume only those dairy products specified in the recommended food list. The types of fats you consume are extremely important and can have a great influence on your overall health.

You also need to pay attention to the amount of pure water and cleansing beverages you're drinking. The goal is a half-ounce of water or other cleansing beverage (raw veggie juice, cultured whey, raw coconut water, or herbal infusions) for every pound you weigh, so someone weighing 150 pounds should drink 75 ounces daily, which is a little more than a half-gallon.

Consuming highly pure, natural spring water or any of the aforementioned "live" beverages is an ideal way to enhance the delivery of nutrients and to facilitate the removal of waste.

MAKER'S DIET REVOLUTION FOODS AND BEVERAGES

Legend: Approved ✓ Avoid ✗

Meat (GreenFinished, wild, pasture-raised, or grass-fed)

✓   beef

✓   veal

✓   lamb

✓   buffalo

✓   venison

✓   elk

✓   goat

✓   bone soup/stock

✓   liver and heart (must be GreenFed)

✓   beef (GreenFed) sausage (no pork casing—natural and nitrite/nitrate-free)

✓   beef (GreenFed) hot dogs (no pork casing—natural and nitrite/nitrate-free)

— — — — — — — — — — — — —

✗   grain-fed beef (conventional or organic)

✗   pork

✗   ham

✗   bacon

✗   sausage (pork)

✗   imitation meat product (soy)

✗   ostrich

✗   veggie burgers

✗   emu

✗   rog

✗   turtle

✗   alligator

Fish (wild freshwater/ocean-caught fish; make sure it has fins and scales)

✓   salmon (sockeye is best)

✓   halibut

✓   tuna

✓   cod

✓   scrod

✓   grouper

✓   haddock

✓   mahi mahi

✓   pompano

✓   wahoo

✓   trout

✓   orange roughy

✓   sea bass

✓   snapper

✓   mackerel

✓   herring

✓   sole

✓   whitefish

✓   fish bone soup/stock

✓   tuna (high fat canned in spring water)

✓   salmon (canned in spring water)

✓   sardines (canned in water or olive oil only)

✗   tilapia (which is often farm-raised)

✗   fried, breaded fish

✗   catfish

✗   eel

✗   squid

✗   shark

✗   avoid all shellfish, including crab, clams, oyster, mussels, lobster, shrimp, scallops, and crawfish

Poultry (pasture-raised)

✓   chicken

✓   Cornish game hen

✓   Guinea fowl

✓   turkey

✓   duck

✓   bone soup/stock

✓   chicken or turkey hot dogs (no pork casing—organic and nitrite/nitrate-free)

✓   chicken or turkey bacon (no pork casing—organic and nitrite/nitrate-free)

✓   deli meats, including chicken and turkey (organic)

✓   chicken or turkey sausage (no pork casing—organic and nitrite/nitrate-free)

✓   liver and heart (must be pasture-raised)

✗   fried, breaded chicken

   ✗   processed lunch meats

Eggs (pasture-raised)

   ✓   chicken eggs (whole with yolk)

   ✓   duck eggs (whole with yolk)

— — — — — — — — — — — — —

   ✗   imitation eggs

Dairy (GreenFed, A1 beta-casein-free, whole milk)

   ✓   Amasai

   ✓   sheep's milk yogurt (plain, organic, and grass-fed)

   ✓   goat's milk yogurt (plain, organic, and grass-fed)

   ✓   GreenFed, raw cow's (with Z protein) milk cheese, sheep or goat milk cheeses

   ✓   whole milk plain goat's milk kefir

   ✓   raw, homemade almond milk

   ✓   coconut milk (organic, free of sugar)

— — — — — — — — — — — — —

   ✗   cow's milk dairy (raw or pasteurized containing A1 beta-casein)

   ✗   goat's milk dairy (unless organic and pasture-fed)

   ✗   sheep milk dairy (unless organic and pasture-fed)

   ✗   soy milk

   ✗   rice milk

   ✗   regular commercial milk, ice cream, or processed cheese food

   ✗   flavored, low-fat, or fat-free cheese, yogurt, and kefir

   ✗   dry milk (many processed foods contain this ingredient)

Fats and oils (organic)

   ✓   flaxseed oil (not for cooking)

✓   pasture-raised butter oil (ghee)

✓   hemp seed oil (not for cooking)

✓   avocado

✓   ghee (clarified butter, organic)

✓   cow's milk butter (organic, grass-fed)

✓   goat's milk butter (organic, grass-fed)

✓   coconut milk/cream (canned or fresh)

✓   extra-virgin coconut oil (best for cooking)

✓   extra-virgin olive oil (not best for cooking)

✓   red palm oil

✓   sesame oil (cold pressed)

✓   peanut oil (cold pressed)

✗   grapeseed oil

✗   lard

✗   margarine

✗   shortening

✗   soy oil

✗   safflower oil

✗   canola oil

✗   sunflower oil

✗   corn oil

✗   cottonseed oil

✗   any partially hydrogenated oil

Vegetables (organic fresh or frozen)

✓   micro greens (hydroponically grown)

✓   squash (winter or summer)

✓ broccoli

✓ asparagus

✓ beets

✓ cauliflower

✓ Brussels sprouts

✓ cabbage

✓ carrots

✓ celery

✓ cucumber

✓ eggplant

✓ pumpkin

✓ garlic

✓ onion

✓ okra

✓ mushrooms

✓ peas

✓ peppers

✓ string beans

✓ tomatoes

✓ lettuce (all varieties)

✓ spinach

✓ artichokes (French, not Jerusalem)

✓ leafy greens (kale, collard, broccoli rabe, mustard greens, etc.)

✓ sprouts (broccoli, sunflower, pea shoots, radish, etc.)

✓ sea vegetables (kelp, dulse, nori, kombu, hijiki, etc.)

✓ raw, fermented vegetables (sauerkraut, kimchi, no vinegar)

- ✓ sweet potatoes
- ✓ corn
- ✓ white potatoes

Beans and legumes (organic and soaked or fermented are best)

- ✓ lentils
- ✓ small amounts of fermented soybean paste (miso) as a broth
- ✓ tempeh (fermented soy bean loaf)
- ✓ natto (a probiotic-infused, fermented soy-based condiment)
- ✓ velvet beans
- ✓ black beans
- ✓ kidney beans
- ✓ navy beans
- ✓ white beans
- ✓ garbanzo beans
- ✓ lima beans
- ✓ pinto beans
- ✓ red beans
- ✓ split beans
- ✓ broad beans
- ✓ black-eyed peas

— — — — — — — — — — — —

- ✗ soy beans
- ✗ tofu

Nuts, seeds, and their butters (e.g. almond butter) organic, raw, and sprouted are best; chew well, especially if not sprouted

- ✓ almonds

- ✓ pumpkin seeds
- ✓ hemp seeds
- ✓ flaxseeds
- ✓ chia seeds
- ✓ sesame seeds
- ✓ sunflower seeds
- ✓ almond butter
- ✓ hempseed butter
- ✓ sunflower butter
- ✓ tahini, sesame butter
- ✓ pumpkin seed butter
- ✓ macadamia nuts
- ✓ hazelnuts
- ✓ pecans
- ✓ walnuts
- ✓ Brazil nuts
- ✓ cashews
- ✓ peanuts (in limited quantities and must be organic)
- ✓ peanut butter (in limited quantity and must be organic)

- ✗ honey-roasted nuts

Condiments, spices, seasonings, cooking ingredients, and salad dressings (organic)

- ✓ ketchup (organic)
- ✓ hot sauce (preservative-free)
- ✓ salsa (fresh or canned, organic)
- ✓ guacamole (fresh)

✓ tomato sauce (no added sugar)

✓ apple cider vinegar

✓ soy sauce (wheat-free), tamari

✓ mustard

✓ Herbamare seasoning

✓ whole mineral sea salt (Celtic, Real Salt, Himalayan salt)

✓ omega-3 mayonnaise

✓ umeboshi paste

✓ Bragg brand salad dressings

✓ coconut aminos

✓ balsamic vinegar

✓ red wine vinegar

✓ herbs and spices (no added stabilizers)

✓ pickled ginger (preservative and color free)

✓ wasabi (preservative and color free)

✓ capers

✓ cooking wine (organic red and white de-alcoholized after cooking)

✓ homemade salad dressings and marinades using MDR-recommended ingredients

✓ organic flavoring extracts (alcohol-based, no sugar added, vanilla, almond, etc.)

✗ all spices that contain added sugar

✗ commercial ketchup with sugar

✗ commercial barbecue sauce with sugar

✗ white vinegar

Fruits (organic fresh, frozen, or dried* and no more than two servings per day, best eaten with healthy fats)

* dried fruit must be sugar- and sulfite-free

- ✓ blueberries
- ✓ strawberries
- ✓ blackberries
- ✓ raspberries
- ✓ aronia berries
- ✓ grapefruit
- ✓ lemon
- ✓ lime
- ✓ cranberries (fresh or frozen)
- ✓ olives
- ✓ green apple
- ✓ pomegranate
- ✓ apples (with skin)
- ✓ melons
- ✓ apricots
- ✓ peaches
- ✓ grapes
- ✓ orange
- ✓ pears
- ✓ papaya
- ✓ kiwi
- ✓ nectarines
- ✓ pineapple
- ✓ plums

✓ figs

✓ cherries

✓ bananas

✓ mangos

✓ dried fruit (sulfite-free)

✓ canned fruit (organic in its own juice)

Beverages

✓ pure, spring water with low total dissolved solids

✓ botanically infused pure spring water

✓ cultured whey beverages

✓ kombucha

✓ kvass

✓ probiotic sodas

✓ probiotic coffee

✓ purified water

✓ coconut water (must be raw)

✓ herbal teas and infusions (preferably organic)—unsweetened or with a small amount of honey

✓ raw vegetable juice (mostly green with beet or carrot juice—maximum 50 percent of total)

✓ certified organic coffee—buy whole beans, freeze them, and grind them yourself when desired; flavor only with organic cream and a small amount of honey

✓ natural sparkling water

✗ alcoholic beverages of any kind

✗ fruit juices

✗   pre-ground commercial coffee

✗   chlorinated tap water

✗   sodas

Sweeteners

✓   honey (raw, unheated is best)

✓   evaporated coconut nectar/coconut sugar

✓   stevia (raw, green leaf and in small amounts)

✓   Lo Han Guo

✓   sugar (organic cane sugar, evaporated cane juice, and organic brown sugar)

✓   maple syrup

✓   sugar alcohol, including sorbitol and malitol, xylitol (in small quantities such as in mints and gum)

✓   agave nectar (must be raw and in small amounts)

— — — — — — — — — — — — —

✗   fructose or corn syrup

✗   all artificial sweeteners, including aspartame, sucralose, and acesulfame K

Grains and Starchy Carbohydrates (organic, soaked or sprouted is best)

Grains such as wheat, kamut, spelt, oats, barley, and rye contain gluten or gluten-like substances and should be consumed in soaked or sprouted or yeast-free whole grain breads.

✓   quinoa

✓   amaranth

✓   buckwheat

✓   millet

✓   brown rice

✓   sprouted cereal

✓   sprouted, Ezekiel-type bread

✓   sprouted Essene bread

✓   corn grits (organic only)

✓   corn tortillas (organic only)

✓   whole-grain yeast-free bread

✓   kamut (must be soaked or sprouted)

✓   spelt (must be soaked or sprouted)

✓   oats (must be soaked or sprouted)

✓   barley (must be soaked or sprouted)

✓   rye (must be soaked or sprouted)

✗   pastries

✗   baked goods

✗   white rice

✗   dried cereal

✗   instant oatmeal

✗   bread (except sprouted or sourdough)

✗   pastas (except whole-grain kamut, spelt, or quinoa and in limited quantities)

Snacks/Miscellaneous (must be organic)

✓   sprouted trail mix

✓   cacao powder

✓   carob powder

✓   healthy popcorn

✓   macaroons (made with simple ingredients and organically sweetened)

THE MAKER'S DIET REVOLUTION: SAMPLE 3-DAY EATING PLAN

Day 1

7 A.M.: cleansing beverage (spring water, herbal infusion, cultured whey, or green juice)

9:30 A.M.: cleansing beverage (spring water, herbal infusion, cultured whey, or green juice)

12 P.M.: cleansing beverage (spring water, herbal infusion, cultured whey, or green juice)

1:30 P.M.: green salad with mixed greens, tomatoes, avocado, carrots, cucumbers, celery, red cabbage, red peppers, and red onions topped with three ounces of canned high omega-3 tuna, two ounces of Raw Cheddar Bites, and one ounce of sprouted sunflower seeds.

For the salad dressing, mix extra-virgin olive oil, apple cider vinegar or Terrain Living Herbals, and high-mineral sea salt, herbs, and spices, or you may mix 1 tablespoon of extra-virgin olive oil with 1 tablespoon of organic store-bought dressing.

3 P.M.: cleansing beverage (spring water, herbal infusion, cultured whey, or green juice)

3:30 P.M.: raw food energy or protein bar

5 P.M.: cultured veggies

5:30 P.M.: GreenFed Meatloaf (see page 262 for recipe)

Mexican Quinoa (see page 253 for recipe)

Garlicky Green Beans (see page 261 for recipe)

6:30 P.M.: cleansing beverage (spring water, herbal infusion, cultured whey, or green juice)

7:30 P.M.: total omega smoothie

Mix the following in a high-speed blender to make a thick, almost pudding-like smoothie. May be frozen for a custard-like dessert.

1 cup plain Amasai or goat-milk yogurt or kefir 1 tablespoon organic raw honey 2 organic pasture-raised eggs (see disclaimer on page 210) 1 tablespoon extra-virgin coconut oil dash of vanilla extract (optional)	1 fresh banana ½ fresh medium-sized avocado 2 tablespoons EA Live Chocolate Almonds (optional) 3 tablespoons Terrain Omega Powder or EA Live Sprouted Seven Blend (add last while other ingredients are blending)

9 P.M.: cleansing beverage (spring water, herbal infusion, cultured whey, or green juice)

Day 2

7 A.M.: cleansing beverage (spring water, herbal infusion, cultured whey, or green juice)

9:30 A.M.: cleansing beverage (spring water, herbal infusion, cultured whey, or green juice)

12 P.M.: cleansing beverage (spring water, herbal infusion, cultured whey, or green juice)

1:30 P.M.: Beef Avocado Salad with Rosemary Dressing (see page 250 for recipe)

carrot sticks

3 P.M.: cleansing beverage (spring water, herbal infusion, cultured whey, or green juice)

3:30 P.M.: raw cheese and blueberries

5 P.M.: green salad with mixed greens, tomatoes, avocado, carrots, cucumbers, celery, red cabbage, red peppers, red onions, and one ounce of sprouted pumpkin seeds.

For the salad dressing, mix extra-virgin olive oil, apple cider vinegar or Terrain Living Herbals, and high-mineral sea salt, herbs, and spices, or you may mix 1 tablespoon of extra-virgin olive oil with 1 tablespoon of organic store-bought dressing.

5:30 P.M.: Lemon Garlic Chicken (see page 263 for recipe)

baked sweet potato

Sautéed Veggies (see page 261 for recipe)

6:30 P.M.: cleansing beverage (spring water, herbal infusion, cultured whey, or green juice)

7:30 P.M.: sprouted cereal

six ounces of Amasai or goat milk yogurt or kefir

9 P.M.: cleansing beverage (spring water, herbal infusion, cultured whey, or green juice)

Day 3

7 A.M.: cleansing beverage (spring water, herbal infusion, cultured whey, or green juice)

9:30 A.M.: cleansing beverage (spring water, herbal infusion, cultured whey, or green juice)

12 P.M.: cleansing beverage (spring water, herbal infusion, cultured whey, or green juice)

1:30 P.M.: green salad with mixed greens, tomatoes, avocado, carrots, cucumbers, celery, red cabbage, red peppers, and red onions topped with three ounces of GreenFed steak, two ounces of GreenFed raw jack cheese, and one ounce of sprouted sunflower seeds.

For the salad dressing, mix extra-virgin olive oil, apple cider vinegar or Terrain Living Herbals, and high-mineral sea salt, herbs, and spices, or you may mix 1 tablespoon of extra-virgin olive oil with 1 tablespoon of organic store-bought dressing.

3 P.M.: cleansing beverage (spring water, herbal infusion, cultured whey, or green juice)

3:30 P.M.: sprouted trail mix

5 P.M.: cultured veggies

5:30 P.M.: Blackened Sea Bass (see page 263 for recipe)

Stuffed Cheez Potatoes (see page 260 for recipe)

6:30 P.M.: cleansing beverage (spring water, herbal infusion, cultured whey, or green juice)

7:30 P.M.: fruit smoothie

Mix the following in a high-speed blender:

1 cup plain Amasai or goat-milk yogurt or kefir 1 tablespoon organic raw honey	2 organic pasture-raised eggs (see disclaimer on page 210) 1 cup fresh or frozen fruit

9 P.M.: cleansing beverage (spring water, herbal infusion, cultured whey, or green juice)

SHOPPING TIPS FOR THE MAKER'S DIET REVOLUTION DIET PLAN

When it comes to following the MDR Daily Plan, changing the way you shop for foods will change the way you eat.

The great news is that with the Beyond Organic online virtual farmer's market, you will be able to purchase some of the world's healthiest foods and beverages from our farms and production facilities and have them delivered directly to your family. As for the foods and beverages that Beyond Organic doesn't offer, you will want to purchase them from health food stores and natural markets as well as progressive grocery stores and, of course, local farmer's markets or even better, local farms.

I wouldn't blame you, though, if you walked into your local health food store and felt totally confused. You may have no idea where to begin, or you don't know how to read the food labels. You may not even be sure that everything in the store is truly healthy for you—and you'd be right about that. Don't worry. I have some advice for you.

First, I highly suggest you ask the staff members at your local health food store for advice and assistance. They are almost always informed, friendly, and eager to help.

Second, after reading this section of *The Maker's Diet Revolution*, you'll become much more comfortable and prepared to visit a health food store or natural grocer in your area. Remember, your guiding principle is to shop for fresh organic fruits, vegetables, beans, and legumes, as well as wild-caught fish, pastured poultry, and eggs.

Our bodies were not designed to operate at optimum levels on all the junk food, fast food, prepackaged food, or any of the genetically modified, antibiotic-laden, and growth hormone-laden foods that most Americans eat today. Yes, organic products do cost more, but organic foods give you a higher percentage of nutrients and a lower amount of residual pesticides, no antibiotics, no growth hormones, no foods made from genetically modified crops, and an opportunity for a healthy body and planet.

If you can't afford or are unable to locate organic produce, however, the next best thing to organic is to apply a vegetable wash to your conventionally grown vegetables and fruits. Keep in mind that it's much better to consume fruits and vegetables than not to eat them, even if they are not organic. That said, many grocery stores are now carrying certified organic produce.

CONSUMING HEALTHY FRUITS AND VEGETABLES

Certified organic fruits and vegetables have an incredible amount of nutrients—vitamins, minerals, live enzymes, antioxidants, and many other beneficial compounds. Depending on what season it is, there are different fruits and vegetables available, but every fruit and vegetable has something unique to offer. Let's take a closer look at some of the healthiest foods on the planet.

Berries such as strawberries, blueberries, blackberries, and raspberries are all high in antioxidants and some of the most important fruits you can consume. Antioxidants are beneficial compounds found naturally in the body and in plants such as fruits and vegetables—especially berries.

As cells function normally, they produce damaged molecules; these are called free radicals. Free radicals are highly unstable and steal components from other cells, including DNA, thereby spreading the damage. This damage continues in a chain reaction, and entire cells soon become damaged and die off. This process can be beneficial because it helps the body destroy cells that have outlived their usefulness. When left unchecked, though, this process can destroy or damage healthy cells. Eating high-antioxidant foods can help the body preserve the health of our cells.

Of course, buying your berries fresh is best, but frozen berries are a great source of antioxidants year round.

Check out these amazing berry benefits:

- Blueberries are prized as a high source of antioxidants with great overall health benefits.

- Cranberries, usually consumed seasonally, are another great source of antioxidants. They are excellent for urinary tract health and come to a harvest peak in November; thus their association with Thanksgiving.

- Raspberries contain ellagic acid, which is an antioxidant with immune-boosting properties and excellent benefits for female health. They are also high in pectin, which makes them an excellent thickener in homemade jellies and jams.

- Pineapple contains bromelain, an enzyme that aids digestion of protein. Eat pineapple fresh or frozen, not canned.

If you eat dried fruits, avoid the kind with sulfite preservatives. Sulfites, or sulfur-based preservatives, are added to hundreds of foods to stop spoilage, but these can be toxic to the human body. Some studies have shown that sulfur additives may contribute to digestive upset. So choose your pineapple and all other dried fruits sulfite- and preservative-free.

Avocado, a much-maligned food, is a fruit, not a vegetable. Avocados contain high-quality fats as well as vitamin E and are a great source of fiber and potassium. Avocados contain monounsaturated fats, similar to those found in olive oil.

Lettuce comes in several varieties and is high in fiber. The more colorful varieties are great sources of antioxidants. Americans are used to consuming iceberg lettuce, but today there are many great mixed green blends. These mixed green blends contain organic baby lettuces, including green oak leaf, organic baby spinach, red and green chard, and arugula. They're pre-washed, and they're easy for people who don't have a lot of time on their hands. These greens contain virtually every mineral and trace element and large amounts of beta-carotene, which fits into the nutritional category of carotenoids, a class of very important antioxidants that give fruit and vegetables their bright colors.

Cabbage is excellent for the digestive tract, particularly when fermented or juiced. It contains something called vitamin U, which is known as the anti-ulcer vitamin. Cabbage is also extremely effective as sauerkraut, making it very bio-available.

Mushrooms are high in nutrients, particularly the mineral selenium, which works with vitamin E as an antioxidant and binds with toxins in the body, rendering them harmless. Mushrooms are over 90 percent water and are high in biotin, one of the B-complex type vitamins.

Mushrooms are one of those foods that should be eaten organically because of where they are grown. Mushrooms pick up many nutrients from the soil and the trees they are grown on. If they are grown in a non-organic environment, however, they are often high in heavy metals, so you want to be careful about eating non-organic mushrooms. Despite what you hear, eating mushrooms does not contribute to yeast overgrowth in the body. Some people who are yeast sensitive, however, have cross-sensitivities to mushrooms and should proceed with caution.

Peppers are rich in antioxidants, which prevent oxidative damage to the body. Green peppers may be more difficult to digest than other colored peppers, so if you have complicated digestive problems, you should eat yellow, orange, or red peppers. The different colors are rich in different nutrients as well. Red peppers are substantially higher in vitamins C and A than green peppers.

Sweet potatoes are one of the highest sources of beta-carotene. Sweet potatoes also contain vitamin C, calcium, potassium, carbohydrates, and fiber.

Eggs contain all the known nutrients except for vitamin C. They are good sources of the fat-soluble vitamins A and D as well as certain carotenoids that guard against free radical damage to the body. They also contain lutein, which has been shown to support ocular health. But please note that when it comes to healthy kinds of eggs, not just any old egg will do.

What kind of eggs should you look for in your health food store? Organic pasture-raised, high omega-3 eggs. They are nature's perfect food. When possible, try to buy eggs from farms where the chickens are allowed to roam free and eat their natural diet. Eggs produced from chickens in their natural environment contain a healthy balance of omega-3 fatty acids to omega-6 fatty acids and DHA, which is good for the brain and eyes. High omega-3/DHA or organic eggs have six times the vitamin E and nine times the omega-3 fatty acids as regular store-purchased eggs.

You have heard that you should watch how many eggs you eat because they are high in cholesterol. The myths about cholesterol are completely unfounded. Eggs can be a healthy addition to anyone's diet. They can be consumed in a variety of ways—fried, hard-boiled, soft-boiled, and poached. Eggs can be used in baking and can even be added to the smoothie recipes found on pages 254-257.

CONSUMING HEALTHY POULTRY AND FISH

I recommend **organic, pasture-raised chicken, turkey, and duck.** When purchasing poultry, look for chicken and turkey that has been raised on a soy-free diet. Poultry is healthiest when consumed in a soup or stock. Dark meat has more nutrients than the white meat.

For seafood, eat only fish with fins and scales caught in the ocean or freshwater lakes and streams, not farm-raised fish. **Salmon, halibut, tuna, cod, sea bass, and sardines** are highly recommended, but don't eat shellfish and crustaceans because they contain abundant toxins from their water-bound scavenging habits. In fact, scientists gauge the contaminant levels of our oceans, bays, and rivers by measuring the biological toxin levels in the flesh of crabs, oysters, clams, and lobsters.

Wild salmon, with sockeye being one of the best varieties, is loaded with healthy protein, omega-3 fatty acids, vitamin D, and the antioxidant astaxanthin, which has been extensively studied and shown to benefit the entire body with its powerful antioxidant effects.

Believe it or not, you can find very healthy seafood in a can. The big key is whether the can is marked "wild caught" rather than "farm raised." You want to choose the former. The good news is that when you are looking for salmon, sardines, and even herring, canned is almost always going to be wild.

High-quality sardines are one of the world's greatest foods, although many people hold their nose just thinking about them. Whole, canned sardines are an extremely rich source of omega-3 fats and contain as much calcium as a glass of milk. Make sure to obtain sardines that contain edible soft bones and organs of the fish, which make it a total package.

I also recommend wild-caught canned tuna, but it would be wise to restrict canned tuna to one or two cans a week based upon their possible contamination with heavy metals and PCBs. Research shows chunk light tuna contains less mercury than other types because the natural oils contained in fish are detoxifiers of heavy metals.

So, when consuming tuna, try to eat chunk light. You can also look for high omega-3 tuna, which is a more premium product coming from younger, fattier fish. Look for tuna canned in spring water with a high amount of fat (6 to 8 grams) per serving. Tuna higher in fats are usually lower in toxins such as heavy metals. The advantage of buying tuna in a health food store is that the product doesn't contain additives or preservatives. The fewer ingredients, the better.

Omega-3 fatty acids—the fats we lack the most in our diet—are critical in negating the effects of the overabundance of omega-6 acids and hydrogenated fats found in the standard American diet. The ratio of omega-3 fatty acids to omega-6 fatty acids can be balanced by consuming more omega-3 foods such as ocean-caught fish with fins and scales (salmon, tuna, and sardines) and eggs high in omega-3 fats.

CONSUMING HEALTHY GRAINS

When on the Maker's Diet Revolution eating plan, you can include grains such as **amaranth, millet, quinoa, buckwheat, and brown rice,** as well as cereals and breads made with sprouted grains. Feel free to enjoy whole organic grain products in your diet as long as they have been properly prepared through soaking, sprouting, or fermenting.

When choosing bread, look for the term "sprouted" on the label. Varieties such as Ezekiel and Essene-style breads are extremely high in fiber and can be very nutritious. You can tell a good whole-grain sourdough bread when the label lists a handful of ingredients such as whole grain spelt, water, and sea salt and has the designation as a "whole-grain yeast-free bread." When you buy bread made from sprouted organic grains or whole grain sourdough bread, you can be assured that you're getting the highest-quality products.

White bread is totally devoid of any nutritional properties and should never be eaten—never. In fact, a diet high in white bread, white rice, and white potatoes puts women at much higher risk of pancreatic cancer, especially if they are overweight and don't get adequate exercise, according to a National Cancer Institute report from 2002.

Whole-grain sourdough and sprouted breads and cereals are healthy grain foods for most people, unless you have a known intolerance to gluten. Before the advent of modern food processing technology, it was common for our ancient ancestors to soak their grains overnight and then allow them to dry in the open air until they sprouted. Many times they allowed their grains to go through an ancient leavening process that resulted in whole-grain sourdough bread.

Be aware that white rice is just like white bread, meaning that it is a high-glycemic carbohydrate that is absorbed quickly into the bloodstream and can raise insulin levels rapidly. As a result, white rice causes a spike of blood sugar and a surge of insulin. Instead, try whole-grain brown or wild rice, amaranth, millet, quinoa, buckwheat, or oats soaked overnight. Instant oatmeal is processed and refined and is much less healthy than slowly cooked whole oats. Puffed or flaked wheat, oats, and rice have been processed by high heat and pressure. They also shoot your insulin levels way up.

Some of the largest sources of mineral-depleting nutrients are contained in the sugary breakfast cereals lining the shelves of America's grocery stores. Studies show these cereals can have even more detrimental effects on blood sugar than refined sugar and white flour.

As a healthier alternative, I recommend hot cereals made from soaked or sprouted whole grains. They are not processed and do not have preservatives, artificial flavors, added colors, added synthetic vitamins, hidden sugars, or artificial sweeteners.

CONSUMING HEALTHY OILS, SPICES, CONDIMENTS, AND SALT

When it comes to oils, I suggest cooking and baking with saturated fats, which are stable, healthy fats. The two best fats to cook with are **extra-virgin coconut oil** and **organic red palm oil.** These fats can withstand high heat without oxidizing.

Coconut oil promotes a healthy microbial balance and supports healthy digestion and immune system function. High-quality extra-virgin coconut oil produced through natural fermentation should have the aroma of a fresh coconut.

Margarine is a man-made fat produced by using bleaching agents, deodorization, and high heat, destroying nearly all of its nutrients. Margarine contains harmful hydrogenated oils. These hydrogenated oils contain trans-fatty acids and are the real culprits behind many of our nation's health problems.

Olive oil is extremely healthy, but olive oil should be used only on food and never heated. Look for certified organic extra-virgin olive oil in a dark bottle since light coming into clear bottles can decrease some of the important health properties of the oil as well as its freshness. Extra-virgin olive oil is produced from the first cold pressing of the olives, and that's where you'll get the most antioxidants and other nutrients. Choose a colorful oil with a rich aroma. Stay away from the hydrogenated vegetable oils and polyunsaturated oils, especially when cooked, as well as soy, sunflower, canola, or safflower oils.

When choosing cooking oil, your first choice should be **extra-virgin coconut oil** or **virgin palm oil**. Since extra-virgin olive oil is not as stable under heat as coconut oil or palm oil, it is best used in salad dressings. Polyunsaturated oils are unstable fats that should not be used as cooking oils. These include flaxseed oil (healthy when used on and in foods, however), canola oil, sunflower oil, corn oil, safflower oil, soybean oil, and cottonseed oil.

Read the labels of the food you buy because fats and oils are frequently key ingredients in packaged foods. Many contain artificially processed fats and oils that are hydrogenated and partially hydrogenated oils that contain trans-fatty acids. The processing they undergo makes them more stable, enabling them to sit on a shelf for years at a time, but this process also makes them damaging to our bodies.

The best spices are organic because they don't contain caking agents and other preservatives that you may find in non-organic spices. Flavored blends are combination seasonings with a variety of organic herbs and spices. Some other favorite seasonings include unrefined sea salt seasonings. You can use them in cooking and add them to your favorite foods.

Cultured veggies and **spicy kimchi** are condiments *par excellence*. Be brave and give them a try. This would also be a good time to clear your refrigerator and pantry of any commercial ketchup, mustard, mayonnaise, pickled relish, or other common condiments. Organic versions of these popular condiments are readily available these days, even in supermarkets. They come without refined sugar and unhealthy preservatives.

Regular table salt is highly refined with chemical and high temperature processes. These processes remove many of the valuable minerals, use harmful and potentially toxic additives, and employ bleaching agents to make the salt pristine white. **Unrefined sea salt**, however, has many important minerals, and can be slightly gray or pink in color. Celtic Sea Salt and Real Salt are recommended brands.

CONSUMING HEALTHY SWEETENERS

We've all seen the pink, blue, and yellow packets on restaurant tables. Stay away from those artificial sweeteners! Aspartame, saccharin, sucralose, and their sweet cousins are made from chemicals that have sparked debate for decades. Though the Food and Drug Administration has approved the use of artificial sweeteners in drinks and food, these chemical additives may prove to be detrimental to your health in the long term. The fear is that these highly addictive artificial sweeteners can cross the blood-brain barrier, causing neurological problems.

The best sweetener to use is **raw, unheated honey**, which is a rich storehouse of naturally occurring enzymes. My second favorite sweetener is evaporated coconut nectar, also known as coconut sugar. Some other acceptable sweeteners are **organic cane sugar** and **organic maple syrup**.

CONSUMING HEALTHY NUTS AND SEEDS

The good news is that snacks have a place in the MDR eating plan. The bad news is that when blood sugar levels fall, many reach for a candy bar or soda for a quick "pick me up." These commercially produced snack foods are loaded with sugar, preservatives, and artificial ingredients that can rob you of your good health.

Some of the most convenient and healthiest snacks are nuts and seeds, which are great sources of fiber, healthy fats, and nutrients. If properly prepared, they are extremely nutritious. "Properly prepared" means raw, soaked, or sprouted. Make sure they are organic. Try **almonds, walnuts, pecans, pumpkin seeds,** and **sunflower seeds**. The most nutritious seeds are **flaxseeds** and **chia** and **hemp seeds**, all loaded with omega-3 fatty acids and fiber.

Raw nut butters made from almonds, cashews, and sunflower seeds are something worth checking out. They're better, in my opinion, because when they're raw—not roasted or heated—they're easy to digest and still have their vitamins, minerals, and enzymes. Nut butters can be used as a veggie dip or spread onto sprouted bread or fresh fruit.

It is worthy to note that the phytates found on the covering of grains and seeds "grab" minerals in the intestinal tract and block their absorption. The sprouting process effectively removes these phytates from the outer covering of the natural grain. Germination initiates a chemical transformation in the seed grains that neutralizes the phytates, causing them to come alive, making all of the nutrition within the seed available for digestion.

Dining Out Tips

I'd like to offer you some tips when you eat out:

1. Opt for water as your beverage of choice, preferably spring or filtered (not chlorinated). Avoid alcohol, juice, and soda and consume only organic tea or herbal infusions.

2. Don't reach for the bread or chips at the table. This includes dinner rolls, bread sticks, sliced bread, muffins, and tortilla chips

3. Avoid appetizers as much as possible. Eat your salad before eating your entrée.

4. When ordering soup, make sure no sugar is added. Avoid the use of toppings such as crackers, croutons, bacon, cream cheese, or cheese.

5. Choose the house salad over the Caesar salad or other salads with numerous ingredients and toppings. The plainer the salad, the better.

6. Salad dressing is real simple—balsamic vinegar and extra-virgin olive oil. Other dressings are full of hydrogenated oils and sugars. It is safer to just order the balsamic vinaigrette as the waiter may not know exactly what is in the other dressings. Also, avoid the croutons.

7. Ask your server how the food is prepared. To avoid some hidden traps in your meal, inquire about the butter, margarine, cream, or oil that may be used in preparing that item. Have your meal cooked in olive oil or butter. Look for the words grilled, poached, baked, roasted, or broiled on the menu.

8. Request that your food be prepared without MSG or sugar.

9. Avoid entrées with a lot of ingredients. Avoid foods that have the following descriptions: fried, buttery, creamy, rich, au gratin, scalloped, béarnaise, Newburg, BBQ, sweet and sour, teriyaki, or breaded.

10. For your main entrée, use the following pecking order when choosing a protein:

    - wild fish
    - wild game (venison or bison)
    - lamb (most lamb is raised well in Australia or New Zealand and fairly well in the States)
    - beef (best if organic or pasture-raised)
    - farm-raised fish (not the healthiest food by any stretch, but still an okay option for dining out)
    - chicken (by far the worst of the biblically clean, conventionally raised animals due to the way factory-farmed poultry is treated and processed)

11. Don't be afraid to make special requests. Most restaurants are willing to accommodate your dietary needs when possible. Order steamed vegetables instead of mashed potatoes, French fries, or coleslaw.

12. There is no need to dress your food up with salt. Most foods already have salt added to them while being cooked.

13. If you order eggs as your main dish, mix it up by requesting diced tomatoes, peppers, and onions—but no ham, please.

14. If you are eating a light dinner, try a salad with grilled wild fish, topped with olive oil and balsamic vinegar for the dressing.

Examples of Clean Meats in the Eyes of God

Meat:

- beef
- antelope
- elk
- buffalo
- lamb
- venison
- goat
- sheep

Fish:

- cod
- haddock
- mackerel
- salmon
- tuna

Fowl:

- chicken
- turkey
- quail
- pheasant
- goose
- grouse
- duck
- guinea fowl

The Maker's Diet Revolution Quick Eating Tips

- Eat only foods that God created.
- Don't alter God's design, which means eat foods in a form that is healthy for the body.
- Don't let any food or drink become your idol.
- Chew each mouthful of food twenty-five to fifty times for improved digestion.
- At mealtime consume protein, fat, and veggies before starchy carbohydrates or sweet deserts.
- Drink six to eight or more glasses of pure water or other cleansing beverages per day and drink eight ounces of water whenever you feel hungry.
- When the food on your plate is half-eaten, take a deep breath and ask yourself if you're still hungry.

19

REVOLUTIONARY RESULTS

One of the great things about putting together a regimen like the Daniel Diet is looking into the happy faces of those who've completed this ten-day, partial cleanse program consisting of foods and beverage similar to what Daniel and his three colleagues consumed centuries ago. Their smiles warm my heart, and their improved health inspires me.

I asked some of the folks who've undertaken the Daniel Diet to share their thoughts, and here's what they had to say:

> It's hard for me to believe this, but I lost 20 pounds in ten days (going from 286 pounds to 266 pounds), and I feel great! What a great kick-start to a healthier way of living. I turned sixty-five this year and retired, so I wanted to get serious about my physical, spiritual, and nutritional health.

> Truthfully, I have struggled with overeating much of my life. The Daniel Diet looked like the answer. Ten days seemed like a long time to partially fast, but I was impressed with the thoroughness of the plan. What was especially appealing to me were the daily prayer times and the evening calls where we could get encouragement, guidance, and ask questions.

> I was surprised that I wasn't hungry. At first I thought the food wouldn't be enough, but by Day 6, I couldn't even finish my meals.

After a week, I was beginning to get concerned because I hadn't really experienced any detox side effects, but those happened on Day 9, when I experienced some side effects from the release of toxins from my body. It finally felt good to know that my body was getting rid of these poisons.

I feel better, look better (in my opinion), and most of all, I'm ready to move forward.

—LARRY P.

I felt better on the Daniel Diet than I did when I ate regularly. I wrote in my journal most days, and spiritually, God has revealed Himself to me in greater ways. I really enjoyed my extra time with the Lord and growing closer to Him, being more sensitive to His voice. God is faithful and always shows up during and after a fast— in His timing.

I found the Daniel Diet easier than other fasts I have done in the past. I didn't have to plan meals. I lost a total of 11 pounds.

—ANTONIA P.

Being a home schooling mom of six, perhaps the greatest blessing was how the Daniel Diet affected my children. They listened in on the prayer calls whenever they were around, and each of them seemed to be drawing closer to the Lord during this time. One of my sons, in particular, experienced a very strong spiritual revival. Not surprisingly, his name is Daniel.

—KATHY W.

During the entire time I was on the Daniel Diet, I did not experience any bloating or other undesirable gastrointestinal problems. This was phenomenal! For me, these have been ongoing problems for years, and I am so grateful for the improvement.

—VITINA F.

I participated in the Daniel Diet primarily for spiritual reasons. I have never fasted for more than one day, but I have never experienced days of being more "centered" on the Lord. To pray three times a day and to commit my days before the Lord was amazing.

—Renee Y.

I experienced great support in stress reduction and a decrease in anxiety during the 10-Day Daniel Diet. I have no more PMS or night sweats, and I am sleeping through the night again, which I haven't done for over twenty years. Many people who know me can see the changes in me.

My caffeine addiction is gone as well as my cravings for sweets. God definitely answered my prayers, and my relationship with Him is richer, deeper, and closer.

—Rochelle S.

The first few days of the Daniel Diet were tough from a mental standpoint. I missed some of my favorite foods such cheese and meat.

I was not hungry at all, however. I thought that I might have a coffee headache, but I did not. I lost 10 pounds on the Daniel Diet, but a friend of mine fasted on water the last three days of the Daniel Diet and lost 18.5 pounds total!

—Dinah T.

I have been on the Daniel Diet for the entire ten days and lost 12 pounds—and I feel great. My blood sugar levels are completely normal!

—Philip C.

I lost 12 pounds on the 10-Day Daniel Diet. Woo-hoo! It was a real challenge, but I'm so glad I stuck with it. I feel much more secure in the weight loss this time around and have a desire to keep going.

—Alice C.

I have done a lot of fasting—one-day fasts, three-day fasts, ten-day fasts and twenty-one-day fasts. I have even been on a forty-day fast, but thank you for introducing me to the Daniel Diet. I want to shout the Daniel Diet out to the world and take as many folks on this journey with me as possible.

On the morning of the tenth day, I had lost 15 pounds! I am now able to see a tightness in my skin, particularly in my neck. I have not experienced this kind of weight loss in such a short amount of time with anything I have tried before. I have a ways to go, but I am ready, willing, and able to stay the course.

—SANDI B.

I am so excited that it is Day 10. I can't believe I did it. The Daniel Diet was, by far, a long and arduous road at times, mainly because of the fatigue and utter exhaustion I felt in the middle of the fast. But the last three days I made it through with energy and excitement. It could be the fact that I was accomplishing something that at first seemed so difficult.

—DANIELLE B.

I lost 13 pounds on the Daniel Diet and feel very excited. This evening, I could not eat much of my dinner. I got full quickly, so I guess I've gotten used to eating until I'm full, whereas in the past I would eat until all the food was gone. This is a whole new start for me, and I'm looking forward to the maintenance times of the Daniel Diet.

—ESTHER D.

Jordan said that the Daniel Diet would not be easy, but it would be simple. I actually found it simple *and* easy! That surprised me. I found the pulse to be filling and fulfilling. In fact, many days I couldn't even finish my food.

I did have a social event to attend on the Saturday night during the fast, but I chose to not even go, so I wouldn't be tempted to eat the goodies! I had only 10 pounds to lose, and I lost 6 pounds, so I declare that a success.

—GLORIE M.

This was one of the most challenging ten days I've ever experienced. The longest I've ever made it on any cleanse was five days and then I would quit. This time around with the Daniel Diet, I made it all ten days!

Before the Daniel Diet, my weight started at 174.8. After Day 10, I weighed in at 164.0. That is almost 11 pounds in 10 days! I feel lighter and my clothes fit better.

My body feels better, and I also have better clarity of mind. Before, I often felt fatigued, had a foggy brain, and felt dizzy, but after the ten days, I have clear thinking, I'm no longer dizzy, and I have more energy.

God did reveal some things in my life during the ten days, too, and I feel He released me from certain sins I have struggled with. Overall, I have a positive outlook and feel excited for continuing my journey to better health.

—AMY W.

I have tried many types of cleanses over the past fifteen years. The Daniel Diet was absolutely the easiest cleanse I have ever done. I celebrate that there was no special grocery shopping to do, no food preparation, no pills to take, no juicing to do. I was never hungry, nor even anxious for it to end.

I even did an extra half day because I didn't have time to prepare a nice dinner to break the cleanse. The spiritual support and group motivation was also a wonderful component, and my email questions were always answered.

—COLEEN M.

Disclaimer: The above testimonials are examples of extraordinary results from those following the Daniel Diet. The results were due to a low-calorie, salt-free diet and proper hydration. The average weight loss reported by over 100 participants was 14 pounds for men and 8.4 pounds for women.

20

MAKER'S DIET MEALS

Joining the Maker's Diet Revolution has never been easier. In this section you will find delicious and nutritious recipes for lunches, dinners, snacks, smoothies, and desserts that you and your entire family will enjoy. When preparing these recipes, it is best to use organic ingredients whenever possible.

If you're challenged in the kitchen or are squeezed for time, I have a bit of good news: if you're eating within a smaller time window of six to eight hours as I recommend as part of the Maker's Diet Revolution, that means you don't have to prepare breakfast!

Disclaimers Regarding Raw Dairy, Raw Eggs, Raw Fish, and Raw Juice

The following are government-issued warnings for the consumption of raw or undercooked foods and beverages.

- Raw milk products may contain disease-causing microorganisms. Persons at highest risk for of disease from these organisms include newborns and infants, the elderly, pregnant women, those taking corticosteroids, antibiotics and antacids, and those having chronic illnesses and other conditions that weaken their immunity.
- Consuming raw or undercooked eggs may increase your risk of foodborne illness.
- Consuming raw or undercooked seafood may increase your risk of foodborne illness.
- Juice that has not been pasteurized may contain bacteria that can increase the risk of food-borne illness. People most at risk are children, the elderly, and persons with a weakened immune system.

Note: I am the founder of Beyond Organic and Garden of Life, and, where applicable, I am recommending these companies' products. Regarding other companies that I recommend, I do so because I consume their products and find them to be of good nutritional quality and taste. Beyond Organic and Garden of Life cannot be held responsible for the quality or claims of these products. Please do your research and consult with your healthcare practitioner prior to starting any new diet or supplement program.

Salads

ORIENTAL CHICKEN (OR SALMON) SALAD

Ingredients

3 tablespoons unpasteurized soy sauce	½ green bell pepper, thinly sliced
2 teaspoons grated fresh ginger	½ red bell pepper, thinly sliced
2 skinless, boneless chicken breasts or salmon filets	1 small or medium cucumber, thinly sliced
5 cups mixed salad greens	1 cup sliced green onions
1 cup fresh bean sprouts	2 teaspoons sesame seeds, toasted
1 cup fresh snow pea pods, trimmed	Oriental Salad Dressing (see below for recipe)

Directions

Combine soy sauce and ginger in a shallow baking dish. Add chicken or salmon. Cover and marinate in refrigerator up to 4 hours. Remove chicken or salmon from marinade and discard remaining marinade. Cook chicken or fish until lightly browned. Comb ine mixed salad greens and next six ingredients.

Pour ½ cup Oriental Salad Dressing over salad and toss. Arrange cooked chicken or salmon on top and pour more salad dressing on top. Serve with Oriental Salad Dressing and yields four servings.

ORIENTAL SALAD DRESSING

Ingredients

4 tablespoons rice vinegar	2 cloves garlic, peeled and mashed
2 tablespoons unpasteurized soy sauce	1 teaspoon raw honey
2 teaspoons grated ginger	⅔ cup extra-virgin olive oil
2 teaspoons toasted sesame oil	2 teaspoons flaxseed oil
2 teaspoons finely chopped green onion or chives	

Directions

Place all ingredients in a jar and shake vigorously. **Makes 1 cup**.

BLENDED RAW ENERGIZER

Ingredients

1 cup green lettuce	½ medium-sized cucumber, peeled and cut into 3 or 4 pieces
1 cup sunflower sprouts	
1 ripe avocado, peeled and pitted	juice of ½ lemon
1 ripe tomato, coarsely chopped	1 tablespoon Terrain Omega or ground chia seed
½ red bell pepper, cored, seeded, and cut into 4 or 5 pieces (optional)	

Directions

Combine all ingredients in a high-powered blender and process until smooth. Makes two to three servings.

CHICKEN SALAD

Ingredients

6 oz. of cooked chopped chicken	chopped onions
1 tablespoon of omega-3 mayonnaise	chopped peppers
1 tablespoon flaxseed oil	chopped celery

Directions

Combine all ingredients and serve over lettuce or on toasted sprouted bread. **Makes one to two servings.**

BEEF AVOCADO SALAD WITH ROSEMARY DRESSING

Ingredients

2 lbs. GreenFed steak, cooked medium rare, cut in strips 3 avocados	3 tomatoes, ripe but firm 1 purple onion, thinly sliced 1 bunch Boston Bibb lettuce, leaves only

Rosemary Dressing Ingredients

2 small shallots 1 clove garlic 2 teaspoons parsley, minced 1 sprig fresh or ½ teaspoon dried rosemary 1½ tablespoons Dijon-style mustard ½ cup lemon juice	2 teaspoons raw, unheated honey ⅔ cup Terrain Garlic or raw red wine vinegar 1⅓ cup of extra-virgin olive oil high mineral sea salt, to taste black pepper, freshly ground

Directions

To make the dressing, crush and chop the shallots and garlic together. Mix these with the parsley, rosemary, and mustard. Stir in the lemon juice and honey and let this mixture stand for 2 hours (this portion may be done in advance and stored in refrigerator). Force the dressing through a sieve into a bowl. Add the Terrain Garlic or red raw wine vinegar. Whisk in the olive oil. Season with salt and pepper, to taste.

Add a portion of the dressing to the beef and stir to coat. (If you are starting with fresh meat, you may also marinate the meat in this dressing before cooking). Peel and chop the avocados and tomatoes. Add the avocados, tomatoes, and onion to the dressed beef. Serve on a bed of Bibb lettuce. **Makes six servings.**

Substantial Snacks

TURKEY AND RAW CHEESE WRAP

Ingredients

organic turkey meat	GreenFed Raw Cheddar Cheese
sprouts	hummus, mayonnaise, or mustard
tomatoes	sprouted tortilla

Directions

Place ingredients in sprouted grain tortilla. Add and spread mayonnaise, mustard, or hummus. Roll up tortilla. **Makes one serving.**

EZ PIZZAS

Ingredients

2 slices sprouted whole grain bread or 1 sprouted whole grain English muffin	GreenFed Raw Cheddar or Havarti cheese
pasta sauce	green onions, thinly sliced (optional)
	sea salt or Herbamare seasoning

Directions

Toast bread or English muffins. Place bread on baking sheet. Spoon pasta sauce over bread. Place onions over pasta sauce. Cut slices of cheese and place over onions. Sprinkle with sea salt or Herbamare and cook in oven for 5 minutes or until cheese melts.

Egg Dishes

BASIC OMELET

An omelet is a great way to start the morning and empty out your fridge of leftovers. Below you will find the basic recipe and some fun variations. To get the most nutrition out of your omelet, make sure you choose pasture-raised eggs high in omega-3 fatty acids.

Ingredients

2-4 fresh eggs, at room temperature 2-3 tablespoons extra-virgin coconut oil	pinch of sea salt

Directions

Crack eggs into a bowl. Add water and sea salt, and blend with a wire whisk. (Do not over-whisk or the omelet will be tough). Melt coconut oil in a well-seasoned cast iron skillet or stainless steel frying pan. When foam subsides, add egg mixture. Tip pan to allow egg to cover the entire pan.

Cook several minutes over medium heat until underside is lightly browned. Lift up one side with a spatula and fold omelet in half. Reduce heat and cook another 30 seconds or so—this will allow the egg on the inside to cook. Slide omelet onto a platter and serve.

Omelet Variations to Suit Your Taste

Mexican Omelet: Add salsa, avocado, and jack cheese to omelet just before folding.

Onion, Pepper, and White Cheddar Omelet: Sauté 1 small onion, thinly sliced, and ½ red pepper, cut into julienne strips, in a little extra-virgin coconut oil until tender. Spread this evenly over the egg mixture as it begins to cook, along with 2 ounces of Raw Cheddar Curds.

Garden Herb Omelet: Scatter 1 tablespoon parsley, finely chopped, 1 tablespoon chives, finely chopped, and 1 tablespoon thyme or other garden herb, finely chopped, over omelet as it begins to cook.

Mushroom Havarti Omelet: Sauté ½-pound of fresh mushrooms, washed, well-dried, and thinly-sliced, in extra-virgin coconut oil. Spread mushrooms and grated havarti cheese over the omelet as it begins to cook.

Starches

GARLIC MASHED POTATOES

Ingredients

4 medium potatoes	1½ teaspoons minced garlic
⅓-½ cup plain Amasai or sheep milk yogurt	Herbamare or salt and pepper, to taste
4 tablespoons butter	

Directions

Peel potatoes. Cut potatoes into large pieces and boil in salted water for 35-45 minutes, or until tender. Drain thoroughly. Mash with a fork. Mix plain Amasai, butter, minced garlic, and salt and pepper. Serve immediately. **Yields four servings.**

EASY SPANISH RICE

Ingredients

4 cups cooked brown rice	3 cups cooked tomatoes (you may use canned)
3 onions, chopped	1 cup grated GreenFed Raw Cheddar Cheese
4 tablespoons olive oil	sea salt and pepper, to taste
6 cloves garlic	¼ cup chopped red or yellow pepper
1 teaspoon mustard powder	

Directions

Brown onions in oil and combine with remaining ingredients. Pour into well-greased baking dish and bake at 375 degrees for 35 minutes. **Makes eight servings**.

MEXICAN QUINOA

Ingredients

1½ cups quinoa	1 tablespoon sesame oil
1 onion, finely chopped	1 teaspoon minced garlic
8 oz. canned diced tomatoes	salt and pepper or Herbamare
1½ cups chicken stock, heated	¾ cup fresh cilantro, chopped
1 cup frozen peas, thawed and drained	

Directions

Heat oil in a large pot over medium heat. Add onion and quinoa. Cook for 8-10 minutes or until lightly browned. Stir in garlic and cook for two more minutes. Add tomatoes and chicken stock and season with pepper or Herbamare. Bring to a boil, cover tightly, and simmer over very low heat for 10-15 minutes. Remove from heat and leave covered for 10 minutes or until all the liquid has been absorbed. Stir in peas and sprinkle with cilantro. **Makes four servings.**

Variation: 1 cup of brown rice may also be substituted for 1½ cups quinoa.

Smoothies

During my health journey, I consumed smoothies one to two times per day with raw eggs. Contrary to popular belief, eggs from healthy, pastured, organic chickens have a very low levels of germs. If the egg has an odor, obviously it should not be eaten. Since germs on the shell cause most of the infections, it is best to wash the eggs in the shell with a mild alcohol or hydrogen peroxide solution or a fruit and vegetable wash for added protection. For those who don't want to consume raw eggs in their smoothies, their use is strictly optional.

TOTAL OMEGA SMOOTHIE

Ingredients

8 oz plain Amasai or sheep milk yogurt	1 tablespoon extra-virgin coconut oil
2 raw eggs (optional—pastured	dash of vanilla extract
organic is best)	1 tablespoon EA Live chocolate
1 ripe banana	almonds (optional)
½ medium-sized avocado	3 tablespoons (1 serving) Terrain Omega
1 tablespoon raw honey	or EA Live Sprouted Seven Blend

Directions

Combine all ingredients in a high-speed blender and blend. Best to add the powdered ingredients toward the end as the blender is going. Consistency will be thick, almost pudding-like. **Makes two servings.**

PIÑA COLADA SMOOTHIE

Ingredients

10 oz. of plain Amasai or sheep milk yogurt	½ fresh or frozen banana
2 organic eggs (optional)	½ teaspoon vanilla extract
1 tablespoon extra-virgin coconut oil	3 tablespoons (1 serving) Terrain Omega or
1-2 tablespoons unheated honey	EA Live Sprouted Seven Blend (optional)
1 cup fresh or frozen pineapple	

Directions

Combine the ingredients in a high-speed blender. **Makes two servings.**

PEACHES AND CREAM SMOOTHIE

Ingredients

10 oz. plain Amasai or sheep milk yogurt	1 fresh or frozen banana
2 organic eggs (optional)	½ teaspoon vanilla extract (optional)
1-2 tablespoons unheated honey	3 tablespoons (1 serving) Terrain Omega or
½-1 cup fresh or frozen peaches	EA Live Sprouted Seven Blend (optional)

Directions

Combine the ingredients in a high-speed blender. **Makes two 8-ounce servings.**

TROPICAL SMOOTHIE

Ingredients

10 oz. of plain Amasai or sheep milk yogurt	½ cup fresh or frozen mango
2 organic eggs (optional)	½ cup fresh or frozen banana
1 tablespoon extra-virgin coconut oil	½ teaspoon vanilla extract
1-2 tablespoons unheated honey	3 tablespoons (1 serving) Terrain Omega or
½ cup fresh or frozen pineapple	EA Live Sprouted Seven Blend (optional)

Directions

Combine the ingredients in a high-speed blender. **Makes two 8-ounce servings.**

BANANA CREAM SMOOTHIE

Ingredients

10 oz. of plain Amasai or sheep milk yogurt	½ teaspoon vanilla extract
2 organic eggs (optional)	3 tablespoons (1 serving) Terrain Omega or
1-2 tablespoons unheated honey	EA Live Sprouted Seven Blend (optional)
1 cup fresh or frozen banana	

Directions

Combine the ingredients in a high-speed blender. **Makes two 8-ounce servings.**

SWISS ALMOND CHOCOLATE SMOOTHIE

Ingredients

10 oz. plain Amasai or sheep milk yogurt	2 tablespoons almond butter
1-2 organic eggs (optional)	1-2 fresh or frozen bananas
1 tablespoons extra-virgin coconut oil	½ teaspoon vanilla extract
1-2 tablespoons unheated honey	3 tablespoons (1 serving) Terrain Omega or
2 tablespoons cocoa or carob powder	EA Live Sprouted Seven Blend (optional)

Directions

Combine the following ingredients in a high-speed blender. **Makes two 8-ounce servings.**

BERRY SMOOTHIE

Ingredients

10 oz. of plain Amasai or sheep milk yogurt	vanilla extract (optional)
1-2 organic eggs (optional)	1 serving (3 tablespoons) Terrain Omega or
1-2 tablespoons of raw honey	EA Live Sprouted Seven Blend (optional)
½-1 cup of fresh or frozen berries (blueberries, strawberries, raspberries, blackberries)	

Directions

Combine all ingredients in a high-speed blender and blend until desired texture. **Makes two servings.**

MOCHACCINO SMOOTHIE

Ingredients

10 oz. plain Amasai or sheep milk yogurt	1 tablespoon whole coffee beans
1-2 organic eggs (optional)	1-2 fresh or frozen bananas
1 tablespoon extra-virgin coconut oil	½ teaspoon vanilla extract
1-2 tablespoons unheated honey	1 serving (3 tablespoons) Terrain Omega
2 tablespoons cacao powder	or EA Live Sprouted Seven Blend

Directions

Combine the ingredients in a high-speed blender. **Makes two servings.**

CREAMSICLE SMOOTHIE

Ingredients

8 oz. of plain Amasai or sheep milk yogurt 4 oz. freshly squeezed orange juice 1-2 organic eggs (optional) 1-2 tablespoons unheated honey	1-2 fresh or frozen bananas ¼ teaspoon vanilla extract 3 tablespoons (1 serving) Terrain Omega or EA Live Sprouted Seven Blend (optional)

Directions

Combine the following ingredients in a high-speed blender. **Makes two 8-ounce servings.**

BERRY GREEN SMOOTHIE

Ingredients

1 cucumber, peeled
1 cup berries, fresh or frozen (blueberries,
    raspberries, blackberries or cherries)
½ apple (with peel on)
3-4 leaves of kale
	30 milliliters Terrain Ginger or
	    Terrain Turmeric (optional)
	½ lemon
	1 avocado

Directions

Cut the cucumber and apple in chunks. Place the cucumber, apple, and berries in a blender and process until smooth. Chop the greens and add to the blender along with the juice of half a lemon, the Terrain Ginger or Terrain Turmeric, and process until smooth. Add the avocado and process until well blended. **Serves two.**

Soups

CHICKEN SOUP

Ingredients

1 whole chicken (pastured)	2-4 zucchini (medium)
3-4 quarts cold filtered water	4-6 tablespoons of extra-virgin coconut oil
1 tablespoon Terrain Ginger or	1 bunch parsley
raw apple cider vinegar	5 garlic cloves
4 medium-sized onions, coarsely chopped	2 inches grated ginger
8 carrots, peeled and coarsely chopped	2 inches grated turmeric
6 celery stalks, coarsely chopped	2-4 tablespoons whole mineral sea salt

Directions

Place chicken or chicken pieces in a large stainless steel pot with the water, Terrain Ginger or raw apple cider vinegar, and all vegetables except parsley. Bring to a boil and remove film that rises to the top. Cover and cook for 12 to 24 hours. The longer you cook the soup, the richer and more flavorful the soup will be.

About 30 minutes before finishing the stock, add parsley. This will impart additional mineral ions to the broth. Remove from heat and take out the chicken. Let cool and remove chicken bones and add meat back. **Makes six to ten servings.**

COCONUT MILK SOUP

Ingredients

1 pound chicken or fish, cut into small cubes	1 tablespoon grated fresh ginger
1½ quarts homemade fish or chicken stock	2-4 tablespoons lime juice
1½ cups coconut milk and cream	
3 jalapeño chilies, diced or ½	
teaspoon cayenne pepper, dried	

Directions

Simmer all ingredients until meat is cooked through. **Makes six to eight servings.**

MUSHROOM SOUP

Ingredients

2 pounds fresh mushrooms	1 piece toasted whole grain sprouted or
2 medium onions, peeled and chopped	sourdough bread, broken into pieces
3 tablespoons extra-virgin coconut oil	sea salt or pepper, to taste
1 quart beef broth	plain Amasai
½ cup Terrain Garlic	

Directions

Sauté the onions gently in extra-virgin coconut oil until soft. Meanwhile, wash mushrooms (no need to remove stems, but make sure they're fresh) and dry well. Cut into quarters. Sauté the mushrooms in coconut oil. Remove with slotted spoon and drain on paper towels.

Add sautéed mushrooms, bread, and beef broth to onions, and bring to a boil and skim. Reduce heat and simmer about 15 minutes. Blend soup with a handheld blender. Ladle into heated soup bowls and serve with plain Amasai. **Yields six servings.**

Snacks

CLASSIC GUACAMOLE DIP

Ingredients

4 avocados, chopped	¾ teaspoon onion powder
1 tablespoon Terrain Garlic	½ teaspoon ground cumin
1½ teaspoons high mineral salt	¼ teaspoon garlic powder

Directions

Mash avocados and combine with remaining ingredients. **Yields two to four servings.**

STUFFED CHEEZ POTATOES

Ingredients

4 medium baking potatoes	⅓ cup healthy butter
extra virgin coconut oil, rubbed on skin of potatoes	¾ teaspoon high mineral salt
pink crystal salt, sprinkled on skin of potatoes	¼ teaspoon ground pepper
⅓ cup plain Amasai	1 cup GreenFed Raw Cheddar cheese

Directions

Wash potatoes, rub skins with oil, and sprinkle with salt. Bake at 425 degrees for 1 hour or until done. Cut potatoes in half lengthwise and carefully scoop out pulp. Add plain Amasai, butter, salt and pepper and beat at medium speed of an electric mixer until light and fluffy. Stuff shells with mixture and top each half with cheese. Bake at 425 degrees for 15 minutes or until cheese is melted.

Recipe courtesy of Mandy O'Neil.

Veggies

GARLICKY GREEN BEANS

Ingredients

4 oz. fresh green beans	⅛ oz. Herbamare or sea salt
1 ounce extra virgin olive oil	1 teaspoon garlic and extra-virgin olive oil

Directions

In a large sauté pan, combine olive oil and garlic. Sauté. Add green beans and sauté. Add Herbamare and sea salt to taste. **Makes one serving.**

SAUTÉED VEGGIES

Ingredients

1 tablespoon extra-virgin coconut oil	½ cup thinly sliced carrots
½ cup onion, thinly sliced	1 teaspoon Herbamare or sea
1 cup mix green and red bell peppers	salt to season veggies

Directions

Sauté veggies in coconut oil, allow cooling. **Makes one to two servings.**

Entrees

GREENFED BEEF CHILI

Ingredients

1½ lbs. ground GreenFed beef	1 can Italian-style diced tomatoes
48 oz. tomato juice	chili powder
1 onion, chopped	salt and pepper, to taste
3 cans kidney beans, drained	

Directions

Brown beef in a skillet. In a large pot, bring tomato juice, chopped onion, drained kidney beans, and diced tomatoes to a boil and then turn down to simmer. Add browned meat after it has been drained. Add chili pepper, salt and pepper to taste. Cook on low for 30 minutes. **Serves eight.**

GREENFED MEATLOAF

Ingredients

1½ lbs. GreenFed ground beef	¼-½ cup plain Amasai
1 pasture-raised egg, beaten	1½ teaspoon salt
½ teaspoon Dijon mustard	½ cup oats
½ cup ketchup	1 cup buttered sprouted whole grain toast
1 finely chopped onion	1½ tablespoons coconut sugar
½ finely chopped red pepper (or green)	

Topping Ingredients

½ cup ketchup	2 teaspoons stone ground mustard
3 tablespoons coconut sugar	½ teaspoon chili powder

Directions

Mix ingredients and bake in loaf pan 1½ hours at 350 degrees. Spoon mixed topping ingredients over loaf the last 10 minutes. **Yields four to six servings.**

LEMON GARLIC CHICKEN

Ingredients

12 tablespoons honey	3 tablespoons chicken broth
12 tablespoons lemon juice	6 garlic cloves, mashed
5 tablespoons soy sauce	4 boneless, skinless chicken breasts

Directions

Mix honey, lemon, soy sauce, chicken broth, and garlic in a shallow baking dish. Set aside ½ cup of the mixture. Prick chicken breasts several times with a fork and place in remaining mixture. Cover and refrigerate at least 1 hour. Remove chicken and discard remaining marinade. Grill over medium heat 10-12 minutes on each side, occasionally basting with reserved ½ cup marinade. **Makes four servings.**

BLACKENED SEA BASS

Ingredients

4 6-oz. pieces of fish, cover completely with blackening spice mix	1 tablespoon dulse flakes
1 tablespoon extra-virgin coconut oil	3 tablespoons unpasteurized soy sauce
2 tablespoons cumin seed, ground	1 teaspoon coconut sugar
2 teaspoons coriander seed, ground	1 tablespoon capers

Directions

Heat cumin seed, coriander seed, and dulse for 1 minute in small fry pan with coconut oil. Add soy sauce, coconut sugar, and capers. Blend well. Marinate fish for minimum 3 hours. Heat under broiler on high. Cook fish 2 minutes on each side. **Makes four servings.**

Dressings and Sauces

AMASAI CUCUMBER SAUCE

Ingredients

2 cups plain Amasai	sea salt and freshly ground pepper, to taste
1 cup cucumber, peeled and diced	add a bit of water to thin to desired
1 cup fresh cilantro, chopped	consistency for a dressing
2 tablespoons fresh lime juice	

Directions

Blend all ingredients in processor using on/off turns until cucumber is well blended. Add a bit of water, if needed, for desired consistency for salad dressing. Season with salt and pepper and transfer to small bowl. This sauce can be prepared 1 hour ahead; cover and chill. **Yields 4 cups or about 12 servings.**

SIMPLE RANCH DRESSING

Ingredients

1 cup healthy mayonnaise	¼ teaspoon garlic powder
½ cup plain Amasai	¼ teaspoon onion powder
½ teaspoon dried chives	⅛ teaspoon pink crystal salt
½ teaspoon dried parsley	⅛ teaspoon black pepper, fresh ground
½ dried dill weed	

Directions

In a small mixing bowl, whisk together all ingredients. Refrigerate for 30 minutes before serving.

Recipe courtesy of Mandy O'Neil.

RED PEPPER ITALIAN DRESSING

Ingredients

¼ cup Terrain Sacred Herbs	½ cup extra-virgin olive oil
2 tablespoons fresh-squeezed lemon juice	½ tablespoon Italian spices
2 teaspoons raw creamy honey	¼ cup Bragg's Organic Sprinkle
½ teaspoon pink crystal salt	¼ cup EA Live Slightly Salted
¼ teaspoon ground pepper	Almonds, ground
½ teaspoon paprika	¼ cup red bell pepper, minced

Directions

Blend first six ingredients in a high-speed blender. Gradually drizzle oil while blender is on low speed. Pulse remaining ingredients to mix throughout. Increase speed to high for only a few seconds to thicken.

Recipe courtesy of Mandy O'Neil.

SWEET MUSTARD DRESSING

Ingredients

½ cup extra-virgin olive oil	3 tablespoons chickpea miso
4 tablespoons Terrain Turmeric	1¼ teaspoon mustard powder
1 garlic clove, minced	½ teaspoon pink crystal salt
3 tablespoons raw creamy honey	¼ teaspoon ground black pepper

Directions

Blend ingredients in a high-speed blender. **Suggested serving: Serve with fresh baby spinach and steamed beets.**

Recipe courtesy of Mandy O'Neil.

Desserts

QUICK SPROUTED APPLE CRISP

Ingredients

4 medium baking apples 1 oz. grass-fed butter 1 oz. purified water	⅔ cup EA Live Cinnamon Raisin Granola 2 tablespoons raw honey

Directions

Preheat oven to 375 degrees. Peel, core, and chop the apples. Place apples in medium-sized pot with water and butter. Cover and cook on medium heat for 15 minutes or until apples can be mashed with a fork to the consistency of apple sauce. Stir in 1 tablespoon of honey. Pour mixture into a medium-sized baking dish. Pour granola evenly over apple mixture and press down with a fork. Drizzle with remaining 1 tablespoon of honey. Bake for 15 minutes. Remove from heat, let cool, and serve. **Makes four servings.**

CREAMY HIGH ENZYME DESSERT

Ingredients

4 oz. plain Amasai 1 tablespoon raw, unheated honey 2 tablespoons Terrain Omega or EA Live Sprouted Seven Blend	½ cup fresh or frozen organic berries

Directions

Mix Amasai, honey, and Terrain Omega and top with berries. **Makes one serving.**

VANILLA ICE CREAM (AMASAI)

Ingredients

8 ounces Amasai (milk and honey flavor) 1 raw egg yolk (optional)	½ teaspoon organic vanilla extract dash of sea salt

Directions

Combine all ingredients in a blender and pour into a bowl or porcelain baking dish. Cover and place in the freezer for 2-3 hours. **Serves two.**

VANILLA ICE CREAM (AMASAI) PIE

Ingredients for Crust

2 cups pecans or walnuts
1 cup pitted dates, soaked in water
  for 5 minutes and drained
¼ cup EA Live Sprouted Seven
  Blend or ground flaxseed
	½ teaspoon sea salt
	½ ounce pure vanilla extract

Ingredients for Vanilla Ice Cream (Amasai)

Triple the ice cream recipe above.

Directions

To prepare the crust, place pecans in a food processor and process or pulse until finely chopped. Add the dates, EA Live Sprouted Seven Blend or flaxseeds, salt, and vanilla and process until mixture forms a ball. Turn out into an 8-inch springform pan and press the mixture into a crust. Chill for about an hour until the crust sets. While the crust sets, prepare the ice cream recipe (be sure to triple the ingredients.)

When the crust has set, pour the ice cream mixture over the crust and place in the freezer for 2-3 hours or until completely frozen. Before serving, top with fresh berries. **Makes six servings.**

CRANBERRY APPLE CRUNCH

Ingredients

3 cooking apples (Granny Smith, etc.) peeled and cut into cubes 1 bag fresh or frozen cranberries 1 cup coconut sugar 1 stick melted butter	extra-virgin coconut oil ⅓ cup honey 2¼ cups EA Live Cinnamon Raisin Granola 1½ cups EA Live Slightly Salted Pecans

Directions

Mix apples, cranberries, and coconut sugar and place in casserole dish greased with extra-virgin coconut oil. Mix melted butter, honey, granola, and chopped pecans and pour over apples and cranberries. Bake in a covered dish for 1 hour at 350 degrees. **Makes six to eight servings.**

BLACKBERRY COBBLER

Ingredients

2½ cups frozen blackberries
1 cup whole spelt flour or sprouted omega flour
½ cup honey
⅓ cup coconut sugar
2 teaspoons baking powder
1 cup Amasai (milk and honey flavor)

Directions

Preheat oven to 375 degrees. Melt ½ stick butter in 8 by 8 dish. Mix dry ingredients with 1 cup Amasai and pour on top of melted butter. Pour 2½ cups berries on top of mixture. Bake at 375 degrees for 35-40 minutes. **Makes two to four servings.**

ABOUT THE AUTHOR

Known as America's Biblical Health Coach, Jordan Rubin is the *New York Times* best-selling author of *The Maker's Diet* and twenty additional health titles, including his recent book, *Live Beyond Organic*. An international motivational speaker and host of the weekly television show "Living Beyond Organic," which reaches over 30 million households worldwide, Jordan has lectured on natural health on five continents and 46 states in the U.S.

Jordan Rubin is the founder of Garden of Life, a leading whole food nutritional supplement company, and has earned doctorate degrees in naturopathic medicine, nutrition, and natural therapies. In 2009, he fulfilled a lifelong dream by starting Beyond Organic, a vertically integrated company specializing in organic foods, beverages, and skin and body care products that includes farming operations on over 8,000 organic acres in Missouri and Georgia.

Jordan resides in southern Missouri with his wife, Nicki, and their three children, Joshua, Samuel, and Alexis.